T0209184

AN INTELLECTUAL'S GUIDE TO DIETING

A Journey to Be One of the Beautiful People

Stephen J. Holoviak, Ph.D.

authorHOUSE®

AuthorHouse™
1663 Liberty Drive
Bloomington, IN 47403
www.authorhouse.com
Phone: 833-262-8899

Published by AuthorHouse 10/05/2020

ISBN: 978-1-6655-0138-5 (sc)
ISBN: 978-1-6655-0137-8 (e)

Library of Congress Control Number: 2020918662

Print information available on the last page.

This book is a work of fiction. Names, characters, places and incidents
are the products of the author's imagination or used factiously. Any
resemblance to actual persons, living or dead, events, or locales is
entirely coincidental. This work is not intended for recommendations
to any specific eating plan or exercise program. Before starting
any diet or exercise program please contact your physician.

This book is printed on acid-free paper.

CONTENTS

INTRODUCTION

The personal journey to self-improvement is deep-seated in all of us. The statistics on the number of people each year who regularly start dieting, quit smoking, and search for the divine in themselves either spiritually or through organized religion is enormous. More astounding is the number who regularly drop off this personal path to self-improvement. I can attest to the dieting part. I have tried just about every diet possible. All succeeded. I lost weight. All failed, as I gained all the weight back and usually added a few more pounds to boot. I have loosely estimated that I have lost and then gained back the equivalent of five starting players on a professional basketball team. The research shows that these diet-induced weight swings are a health hazard in and of themselves. A good deal of reading and study shows that my piecemeal approach was not the path to self-improvement with the most success.

So what is the "path"? That is what this book examines and hopefully with a bit of embellished humor while still being helpful. The overall concept is that for me it needed to be a 360-degree approach, with a plan to work on many aspects of self change and personal reinvention at the same time or in some combination to include them all along with a better diet. Meaning, how and what we eat, exercise, think positively about life, and participate in spiritual/religious disciplines to name a few all impact lasting results. As an example, a ladies makeover doesn't just involve new lipstick! No, it is more than just that single item. It is a combination of events and efforts, such as wardrobe, facials, massage, you get the idea. The notion put forth here is that a total acceptance of change will achieve the weight-loss goal as a by-product of the 360-degree approach.

This book relates various tales about my self-imposed journey. And, while humorous, they are true. While the tale seems to give the impression of a continuous flow of activity in a small time frame, it really evolved over decades of discovery. As in all storytelling, there is exaggeration for both dramatic and humorous effect—used in recounting some really ridiculous events I encountered on my way to hopefully become "one of the beautiful people." In addition, the book is not designed to be a recommendation for any specific eating regime or exercise program. Any such plans should include the input of your health care providor.

Beautiful is not to be defined as limited to strictly physical looks, as you will see. The story evolves into an approach that offers success on many personal levels beyond weight loss. A discipline regularly suggested is mindfulness. It's about being present and aware of all the chosen aspects that will not only help reinvent oneself but also provide a platform for making better choices.

CHAPTER 1

Reflections: The First Experience

From everything I had read and come to believe, I should have been feeling like a new or reinvented person. Vegetarian eating had all the statistics in its favor. But as I lay in what the guests lovingly referred to as "Camp Granola's" sick bay area, it was anything but a good feeling. I believed my problem was a heart attack brought on by the food. The nurse was struggling to contain a laugh. I reflected back on how my current situation had played out.

The goal was honorable. Go to Camp Granola institute and learn tai chi from a Chinese master instructor. I was taking the big first step toward reinventing myself for a new life of awareness. It would be a life of meditation; tai chi; vegetarian eating; and, drum roll please, seeing life as the special people saw it—those people who appeared to me to have followed this path. After all, they were all fit looking, witty, admired, and seemed to know everything. What was a reason not to emulate them?

My vegetarian transition was to take place at the camp. Back then, vegetarian food was the only cuisine the camp served. It was a forced choice to help a person like me, someone with a lifetime of failed dieting, commit to a new eating habit that would stick. Since then the facility has expanded the eating options.

The personal journey of self-improvement is deep in all of us. The yearly statistics on how many people regularly start dieting, quit smoking, and search for the divine in themselves via a spiritual path or through organized religion is huge. More astounding yet is the number of them who drop off of their special paths to self-improvement. I can raise my hand as to the dieting part. I have followed just about every diet possible; the number of fad diet books I have paid for may well equal the down payment on a nice auto. All succeeded— I did drop the weight, but the weight loss was only fleeting. I refer to them as fads but not in a negative way. Each one I embarked upon was popular at the time. Many are still thriving today. They are sound both in research and as a basis for weight loss. But I needed more than any one eating approach for me to succeed.

Okay, what is the correct path to join the beautiful people? What finally worked is a 360 degree notion to focus attention on several key issues at once or in some combinations which will eventually include all of them. The key areas cover: what we choose to eat, a regular physical exercise routine to follow, positive reframing of life's challenges, and a spiritual component to life. Looking at these areas it becomes clear that a campaign to focus attention on all of them will reinvent the individual. It did for me.

My work in the consulting world and directing programs of significant change for the employees of various organizations involved a similar approach. It is a very similar notion for the individual. A mere declaration of the new way to think about work, customers, suppliers, and ourselves on the job rarely succeeds. Instead it requires a total 360-degree look at our organizations work world. This means a big culture change. The same approach is necessary for a single person to enact everlasting personal change.

My approach to change in these key areas often comes across in a humorous fashion. In retrospect, they are funny. But, at the time and living the confusing journey to change the incidents did no alwayst make me want to laugh. Change is difficult for the majority of people. At times, it was hard for me to keep from feelings of self-pity and depression with the mistakes and failures change often produced in the process.

So, back to the story of Camp Granola. This story dates way back to my first visit there at the very beginnings of my journey on the path.

All in all, my first tai chi class went well-ish. There was no doubt in my mind this was part of the change path. In preparation for coming to Camp Granola, I simply didn't eat the meat portion of my meals for a few days. In retrospect, that was far less than adequate preparation. But my vision of vegetarian eating at that time was that it is was the same as normal eating but sans meat. What a miscue!

The first morning I was late getting up and missed eating breakfast. The 6:00 a.m. meditation and yoga before breakfast was a schedule I was ill equipped to meet. I did better as the week went on. So by lunch I was starving. The smells in the dining hall were great, and my taste buds were in overdrive. To my delight, on the food bar, I spotted oatmeal with brown sugar—yes— two bowls for a starter. Still a bit hungry and maybe a bit venturesome, I spotted something called miso-based soup. It smelled good. Although I wasn't sure what miso meant, I went ahead and had a big bowl. It was a bit salty, but I figured it would replace the loss of salt in my body from the four-hour tai chi workout.

Later in the afternoon, it started. A burp here and an acid stomach buildup there. I popped a Tums or two in my mouth figuring all would be fine. Wrong— very wrong. I began to bloat up to where it was hard to do some of the tai chi bending positions. By evening, the pain was incredible. At this wonderful place of the beautiful people, I felt I would pass to the great beyond without experiencing being a real vegetarian or achieving enlightenment.

Was it an indigestion-induced heart attack? Ergo, my lying in the nurses' sick bay. I went there seeking help. The staff explained the chemistry that my body had produced was in response to a mix of sugar from the oatmeal and the miso ingredients. Not all people get that reaction—probably because they somehow inherently know better. Or their digestive tracks are stronger. I was producing enough gas to delight any utility.

I cried out to the nurse, "Why there are no warning labels that read, 'do not mix'? The food line needs these!"

The nurse smiled and stroked my head gently. She asked if this was my first adventure into vegetarian eating. I confessed it was—like it was not obvious. But I appreciated her gentle handling of my ignorance. I spilled out my heart and soul to her—sort of a lonely and depressed man's deathbed confession. I spoke of my dreams of being one of the beautiful people who display an inherent sense of knowing. I wanted the meditative, environmental auras and the vegetarian, athletic looking bodies this group of people seemed to possess.

I continued to sob, as I wanted to break from a life of steak eating, potato loving, and wine gulping. I wished to transcend into a sense of a higher being. Oh, would my heritage hold me back? Eastern European drinking and eating habits seemed a big obstacle to overcome.

This angel, clad in nurse's garb, smiled and said there would be others.

My eyes suddenly became alight with excitement as I tried to raise up on my elbows. "Spiritual guides are coming to help me?" I asked.

Another smile. "No," she said, "just other would-be

veggies like you who eat wrong. They will also be sharing this room all week."

In the morning, I made my way back to my own room to get ready for tai chi class. I shaved and cleaned up. I knew the past experience had made me a wiser man. Feeling somewhat spiritual from the gravity of my experience, I stopped by the Zen meditation hut for lessons on the way to breakfast. Wow, such a vision—a dozen people all sitting in a lotus position on a *zafu* and *zabuton*. The Zen monk began by offering instructions. Although I felt thinner because of my stomach not bloating, I still could not do better than a half lotus. I rationalized that it was a start.

As I walked to breakfast, I decided it would be conservative choices this morning. There on the food line I spotted something I knew. They looked like Cheerios. A big spoon full of raisins on top of a big bowl of this cereal for starters. It was a leisurely meal with my tablemates. We had really deep discussions.

I was excited and in my mind I yelled, *Oh, which path to follow and vision to seek? Am I on the beginning of the spiritual path?* Here I was eating veggie food, talking deep, and getting ready for tai chi in the mountains!

The warm-ups for tai chi class were helpful. We lay on our backs and raised one knee to our chins and then the other. I shook with fear at what discomfort I'd cast on those around me yesterday during these warm-ups.

Smiling confidently, I stood up and realized something seemed amiss. My stomach swirled in pain. Could this be an appendix attack? Oh no. It appeared

I'd discovered the power of bran. Yes, I was to learn later that the little round Cheerio-ish cereal was pure oat bran! I had done a perfect pivot from what I'd learned in class yesterday—only I knew this was not an idle move.

The situation was getting desperate. The toilet was across an area the size of a football field with just an open grassy area to travel to another stand-alone building. My days as a high school football player kicked in. I bulled through the even lines of tai chi participants and out the door. I was a man with a mission and only a short time frame for success.

Into the building I flew. I hoped the cute environmental figure on the door meant it was the men's room. Split second decision-making was needed. There was another man heading for the stall. I faked left and shouldered him out. In retrospect, I am embarrassed by that move, but truth be told I would have used a forearm shiver to get that stall.

The walk back across the field to class was much more civilized. It gave me the opportunity to reflect on my goals. I had been actively reading books on new age understanding. And I'd even subscribed recently to several magazines I felt would complement my intellectual growth, like a runners' magazine, The *Vegetarian Times*, *Garbage*, and *Mother Jones* to name a few. Check the boxes there. I was now taking tai chi. I'd started the meditation classes here. And, to top it off, I was training and interacting with a famous Zen monk. Phew! It had to be just a matter of time till I had that confident sense of being that everyone else here seemed to have. It would be nice to not be anxious about everything I did here and feel out of place.

Well, I was back and active in the lessons. I was working on the correct way to be in the various positions in the "short form."

It was about an hour later when I sensed again I would need to be leaving. This time I used better judgment and calmly left the room. I am sure this more dignified and calm approach was to the delight of those I'd hurriedly ran past earlier.

I went back to my room, as it had become a toilet vigil. I read some poems by the philosopher Kahlil Gibran, hoping to keep my "on-the-path" progress during my time of distress. It seemed to me to be a dangerous world out there trying to be a cool vegetarian. I questioned whether this aspect of my plan would fail.

Hours past, I lay on my cabin floor, somewhat dehydrated and a bit dizzy. My bodily fluids had been flushed to some distant mountain septic tank. It was dark by now. I still was lying there with my eyes fixed on the door. It seemed so far away and unreachable now.

It was—yes—it was opening slowly. A vision in light was there. Was this a hallucinogenic response from my lack of magnesium? Or perhaps my recent reading of Gitanjali, a book of poems by Nobel poet Rabindranath Tagore and morning meditations had combined to produce this vision? I held out my hand and cried out to God.

God it was not. But a close second. That same wonderful nurse had been informed of the symptoms and my behavior and had come by to check on how I was doing. She helped me up. Arm in arm, we headed toward the food hall with a stop for Imodium AD on the way. She was correct. Dinner and fluids would help me.

I was weak and confused. Good food and deep conservation would restore me to my old self. But I was here to rid myself of the old self. That bit of inner dialogue reassured me of the correctness of my reflections of being on the path.

As I walked down the food bar, tears welled up in my eyes. On no, my worst fears. I recognized nothing. Didn't these professional vegetarians ever eat recognizable food sans meat, like cheese and other stuff? Everything was shaped funny, even though it all smelled great. But good smells had tricked me twice before.

The nurse noticed my anxious state and took me to a chair. She was calm and helpful I senced a charisma about her personality as she took charge. She went into the kitchen. I sat with my hands grasped around a glass of water. About to sip it, I noticed it bubbled. How in the world did vegetarians make plain water bubble? Was nothing safe here? I would recommend the camp issue directions about eating—that is, along with a contribution to their nursing staff.

Truly these enlightened people were amazing. The person sitting next to me at the table explained the carbonation of spring water. I was relieved but did not drink it. The prospect of consuming transformed water overwhelmed me.

The nurse emerged from the kitchen. She was carrying what looked like white light in her hands. I had recently read of white light. Wow, a cosmic experience for dinner. The person on the other side of me explained it was just a shiny ceramic plate. The nurse again stroked my head and said it was just a plain potato with only salt and pepper—three things I recognized.

But I quickly answered that this was no such plain potato. That potato at that moment in time became a vision of beauty and great taste. I think this was my first true experience of being "in the moment," and it was all about a potato.

I ate with passion and delight. As my strength and sanity returned, I began to talk openly with my table partners about my mission to become an enlightened person—preferably vegetarian, though my successes to date were not promising. After some chuckling, several at the table confessed to not always knowing what they were eating and also using heavy doses of liquid Tums. I felt relieved. There was hope. No, it seemed they had not all been born with knowledge or with some special preferred DNA package.

The rest of the week progressed uneventfully, bolstered by the help of fellow tai chi students so I would not miss more classes.

I was examining my successes and failures this week in my goal to become a member of the beautiful veggie humans. Admittedly, I was a bit unsure of myself. I felt this was something that could be learned and that there were many adventures in store for me on this journey to achieve my dream state. My next plan to grow was to register for a retreat program at a Buddhist monastery. Maybe that could be the breakthrough experience I needed?

Being "in Vogue" Is a Temporary Thing

A word of caution about self-reinvention. Do not confuse this goal with being in vogue or cool, as it was referred to when I was twenty something. Yes, the two are quite different, and those who pursue this path often find their lives wrapped up in self-indulgent activities.

When I was a teenager, playing the guitar was definitely "in," especially if you could sing and play folk songs. I bought an old guitar and practiced mightily. But with a mild fine motor disorder, I found that picking the strings for individual notes was out of the realm of possibility. Playing was limited to about five cords, which somewhat ruled out the folk genre for the most part. Singing was never a strong suit, but with the guitar playing loudly enough, I figured it could easily equal Arlo Guthrie in sound pleasure.

Dress is another area of making a statement about being "in." The fashion industry counts on this, with endless fashion changes that many follow with willing purchases up to their credit card limits. The fads were fun in retrospect—to wear or not wear socks, the regular changes in the width of men's ties. I listened to my early mentor where I worked at Merrill Lynch as a young broker, who told me to keep the old-fashioned ties, as they would return. He was correct. I simply sorted through and brought out the new style on the tie rack, dry-cleaned the old, and stored them for later use.

But the most fun came with men's underwear. In my generation, boxers were the only option. Well, the fashion industry developed men's briefs, or tighty-whities as they were euphemistically called back then. The drama broke out in high schools where administrators feared the tight fit over men's testicles would incite reactions among young boys with their emerging testosterone levels. What stopped all the talk aboutnew rules for boys underware in school was the tricky detail of checking what the boys were wearing? It seems no one wanted the job of peeking down the young boys' trousers to find out.

There are countless examples that could be offered. But the point is again showing that following fads is not a path for the transformation of self. Looking nice and presentable is not to be vilified. Just don't get carried away with the notion. Of course, the secondary goal of weight loss is completely lost in the vogue pursuit.

So, with that lesson in tow, the next item on the agenda was to examine traditions that could strengthen the spiritual nature of self. Visiting a Zen monastery seemed a good choice.

There were many options for this on the East Coast of the United States—not to mention flying out to either California or Colorado. I chose one in driving distance.

Some Possible Readings

While writing this and asking others for constructive criticism and helpful ideas, a very good suggestion regularly emerged. It was to include some interesting additional books, magazines, and articles to read for a deeper understanding of the material in each chapter. As this is somewhat of an intellectual's look at both dieting and personal self-reinvention, the idea did fit. Below are a few readings that may be of interest. These chapter-ending recommendations are not intended to be an exhaustive literature search. That said, if any reader wishes to make a case for another addition, please send it, and it can be included in further editions or printings.

Chen, William C. C. *Body Mechanics of Tai Chi Chuan*. 1973.
> This is the book given by William Chen when I went to Camp Granola, and he was the instructor. He is a decedent of one of the original Chinese families responsible for the emergence of tai chi chuan. He is considered a grand master of this martial art.

Liang, T. T. *T'ai Chi Ch'uan: For Health and Self Defense*. New York: Vintage Books, 1977.
> T. T. Liang is another tai chi master, and his is an excellent book not only for the moves and positions but also the philosophy behind the martial art.

Cohen, Kenneth S. *The Way of Qigong: The Art and Science of Chinese Energy Healing.* New York: Ballantine Books, 1997.

Kenneth Cohen is a master teacher of Chinese healing energy and its various forms like qigong and Tai Chi. I studied with him at a retreat center much like Camp Granola, and he used this particular book. I so enjoyed the reading and the depth of every explanation, which even includes the cultural aspects of the Chinese that influenced the growth of the science. For people who love intricate bits of data woven into explaining the forms and positions, this is a great choice to study.

CHAPTER 2

Visit to a Buddhist Monastery

My goal at this point in my life was personal transformation—a sort of reinvention of self. And I believed the total reinvention would carry with it desired weight loss to a healthier level. True, I also secretly wanted to be one of the "all-knowing," slender, fit, population who always eat correctly—apparently vegetarian.

Well, my plan of change called for me to visit a Buddhist monastery. My readings and discussions on Buddhism seemed to offer a philosophy that was flexible yet disciplined in the areas I felt the need for change.

It was not a far stretch for me to seek knowledge via Buddhism. A big chunk of my very young formative years were spent in the Orient, with the majority in Japan. My father believed that, if we as a family were to live and spend significant time in another country, then we should immerse ourselves in that culture. As such, we lived in a Japanese home in Yokohama, and after some mastery of the language, I briefly attended a Buddhist-run monastery school for children.

I must note that my sisters were not subject to the immediate language training and were not sent off to study in a monastery. Back then I believed it a form of parental love preference, with myself on the lower end of the spectrum.

The brief stay there, however, was wonderful. And over the years, I have come to cherish that experience. So my choice of Buddhism on this adult transformational path is partially directed out of comfort from very positive childhood memories.

Secondly, the food served at the monastery is vegetarian and vegan. Plus, the new exposure to alternate meditation forms will be available as well.

I drove to the monastery with an almost lifelong friend. It was a beautiful summer day, and the forecast called for great temperatures and sunny skies throughout the whole visit. We were on PA I-81 motoring along in my soon-to-be classic 1984 Porsche 944. We were both wondering about the wisdom of taking this car to a retreat that would focus on life's simple pleasures and where the bulk of the program would be conducted in the outdoors communing with nature's basic abundant gifts.

My friend remarked that renting an old 1960's VW van would have been just about impossible. I smiled at the reality that we both may be a *bit* out of touch for this experience.

Most of my life I'd confronted the inward feeling that I did not belong in situations where I so much wish to be accepted. That was very clear at my last outing at Camp Granola. I had persevered and would return there again. But why the initial fear? It could well be that much of my intestinal distress had been simple massive anxiety. The "beautiful" people never seemed to suffer this malaise—or so I currently believed.

My friend and I had previously attended a weekend retreat with Thich Nhat Hanh, the famous Buddhist teacher and leader of the Middle Way practice of Buddhism. The middle way means that the extreme fringes and rigidities are replaced by a gentle acceptance of practice. His explanation of this was via the example that dealt with the notion of bowing that is so often seen in Eastern philosophies. His point is, if you want to bow to another, then know why you are choosing this. Do not choose to bow just because it is what is always done.

I was taught as a grade school boy that Buddhism is not any special teaching but, instead, is the way we are as humans. That translates as the way we show our respect for the Buddha or God is the flow of love we extend to our fellow humans.

I learned to meditate as a child in the Orient but must confess that my practice was more than a bit rusty, and this trip would help me rekindle the love of my meditative practice.

As an aside, later years in time, I would study "Christian meditation" and was privileged to teach this practice to several Christian groups.

The ride was scenic even during the initial I-81 and I-84 routes. PA I-84 highway is along the very top of the Appalachian Mountains in central Pennsylvania. What great vistas there are in this remote region of the otherwise densely populated world of the Mid-Atlantic and Northeastern part of America.

Over the years of driving this part of the highway, I had observed nature retaking the large almost mountain-size coal dumps and waste piles. Now, many had green ground cover and trees reaching for the sun. Nature is amazing.

We left on this journey from my historic hometown of Chambersburg, Pennsylvania. That town is filled with interesting history and contains both lush forest and fertile farmlands. As we left I-84, the route selected was mostly two-lane country roads in rural New York State. We skirted New York City in favor of this pleasant option. The monastery was about an hour and half north of the city. The first half of the trip was the same as the drive to Camp Granola Institute.

As we neared our destination, the monastery sat atop a hill in lovely pastureland and was bordered by strong creeks capable of being canoed. We would experience the canoeing tomorrow, late morning. Now, we entered the building and headed to our registration area and then to drop our bags. The first meeting with the monks would be yet this afternoon.

The setting; the building; the monks; the beautiful, knowing other attendees—all seemed perfect. But now I was lying flat on my meditation mat at the first general meditation session, which included all the attendees at this program. Unlike the others sitting in the large meditation circle, I had the most painful charley horse I had ever suffered in my right calf.

While most of the monks were not sympathetic, there was one very sympathetic monk who explained that the probable cause of the pain was from the five-hour drive here and, in a relatively short time after that drive, being sitting cross-legged on a mat for hours. I was grateful to him and agreed that was a contributor. But I knew it was also a combo of too much arthritis and that feeling of I-do-not-belong-here anxiety syndrome that plagued me constantly on this path I had chosen.

I massaged the charley horse, and the nice monk had me move to a chair in the outer circle of the group. To my relief, there were several others sitting on similar wooden chairs. The pain subsidized and my attention returned to the meditation practice of centering.

The specialty of the monastery was communing with nature. And it offered many programs that allowed for this direction. My friend and I had chosen the canoe trip. While much of the visit time was spent with the canoe trip, the first day and a half were techniques of canoeing and philosophy lectures, and the last two days were back in the monastery building again with reflection and lecture. The middle part was spent paddling. The canoe trip was also a camping trip accompanied by several monks. The monks would lead our meditation sessions on the trip.

The food was vegan, which fit the basic pursuit of my goal. Only at this monastery, the attendees actively participated in cooking and cleanup. For those, like myself, who do not know much about vegan cooking this would be very helpful—working along with the paid kitchen cooks as well as some well-informed participants.

My individual attempts at vegetarian cooking at home were off to a tough start. At first it was just sans meat. Then I got a cookbook for vegan/vegetarian use. Well, I had none of the ingredients called for in most of the recipes. To be honest I had never heard of them before. Yes, ingredients from India and China or Japan were common. What further complicated my vegan cooking was living in a small town where the food shopping was fine if there were no special needs, like being a vegan. I mean, in a small town and not near a metro area, I found none of these ingredients. But learning to shop was another adventure to be shared later.

The food provided to us by the monastery staff was simple but good. That said, my first attempt at using a bread maker at the monastery was not the success I'd hoped for. I tried to claim the result was a "flat" black bread.

Based on my difficult first eating experience at Camp Granola, where I was hoping to learn tai chi, I was wiser now about what I selected. Be wary, fellow travelers on the path. Good smell alone is not enough to base a meal selection upon. For this experience, I would basically be living on black bread and oatmeal. The thought of being with intestinal distress while trapped in a canoe was sufficient to limit choice.

Dinner the first day was late evening the same day after suffering "the charley horse incident" in the earlier meditation session. Other than my cramp it had been a wonderful experience up to that point.

No one else, of course, had any similar extreme physical difficulties. But after dinner I gathered with fellow participants to have tea and "talk deep." Yes, I had the need to feel that sense of conscious awareness expansion so lacking in my normal life. The conversations were a chance for me to ask those difficult questions about the meditation visions I had been experiencing. Were they real or just hallucinations from hours of mild arthritic pain while sitting cross-legged?

Everyone seemed to have insights. I do not know where they get their insights from. I must have been living my life in a mental vacuum tube.

It was time to sleep. It was clear that sleep would be a euphemistic notion. The options were either on a straw-like mat on the floor or on a rope bed that looked like a more stable backyard hammock.

Morning came early—especially when it seemed I had just gone to sleep. I was getting the idea that all eastern notions—from tai chi to yoga and meditation— seem to start very early in the a.m. My guess was the rock-hard beds promoted getting up early to escape the lower back pain. Here, we were to be up, dressed, and already cross-legged on a mat by 6:00 a.m.

But first, I had to get off the sleeping mat on the floor. Embarrassing as it was, I needed help standing. My back felt like every muscle was locked in place. I shook my head in disbelief. To achieve this goal on my path of change, I needed to crawl to the nearest wall for support while raising myself to a standing position.

How did these people around me just hop up? Some were in their seventies. I knew it must be the magic brought on by the diet. Yes, the diet, I deduced. It would lead to a leaner, fitter, and suppler body—which then would lead to "insight." I was nodding my head in self-talk confirmation. It was becoming clear that I must keep going with this goal of the vegetarian diet. Yes, I would stay in the moment and not falter because of the stiffness and pain of waking up.

Morning meditation passed without my interrupting the session. Thank God. I felt that was at least a moral victory for those of us new to the path. Despite not disrupting the session, I still had this sense of not belonging. A fear coursing through my brain was that, at some random point, the monk in charge of the teaching would look over my way and ask me a question, and I would present this ridiculous look on my face of total anxiety and confusion in response. So, I never made eye contact.

As it turned out, that was the correct thing to do with a sensei. My whole life in America had been spent learning not only to make eye contact but also to read the other person's body language at the same time. Of course, the beautiful people would be a part of something so different and seem to inherently be aware of the eye contact thing. I now knew that I had to read a cultural guidebook before any other similar trips.

Breakfast here was not a buffet but a limited choice of items on our own table. There was homemade yogurt, black bread toast, and assorted dried and fresh fruits to eat alone or with the yogurt. I chickened out and stuck with black bread toast. It was canoeing later in the morning, and that meant taking no chances with food issues. Although I must confess about wondering how long my body could function on non-fizzy water and plain black bread.

My tablemates were delightful and very helpful. I ventured a question with heavy guarding and disclaimers on my part so as not to sound closed-minded. I was curious why so many Jewish persons were present at the monastery.

Again, my question brought a chuckle from tablemates. It was not, as I'd speculated, that it was a special temple visit. The monk at our table chimed in that they were affectionately referred to as "Jew Boos" (Jewish Buddhists).

I must have looked mystified. Over the next half hour of conversation, the monk and other canoeing-expedition people explained that Buddhism had many Jewish participants who were on their own spiritual paths.

Good grief, I was not alone. While different in our

individual end goals, we were sharing the same highway to get there. It was comforting, and I did gain much insight from them. My knowledge of the Jewish faith was primarily book deep—they added much personal texture to my understanding beyond the just reading. And for me, their faith became more than the basic Wikipedia-level information.

After breakfast, it came time for the canoeing lessons and canoe safety instruction. I was not a canoeist—had done some kayaking. While a kayak is more difficult to get into, it was more difficult to upset or turn over than a canoe. Why mention this? Well, I was not the first one to roll unceremoniously out of the canoe and into the ice-cold pond. No, our monk guru and guide was first. It gave us all a good laugh while we lifted the 90-pound Asian gentlemen out of the water. My guess was, with the wet robes he wore, he weighed considerably more. When he returned in dry clothes, they were not like his prior robes but normal outdoor wear.

After lunch, we loaded our gear and launched into the stream to begin our journey. We paddled and chatted. It was great for me to listen to the monk's insights and have him explain the more intricate differences between Zen, Tibetan, and Vietnamese Buddhism. It was like a private tutoring session where I could ask many questions without tipping my hand to the whole group about my gaps in knowledge. Plus, it was helping rid that feeling of not belonging here. I liked the paddling.

The portages where we had to exit and carry gear

and canoe were not so fun. All this, in basically the morning.

We stopped later just before dusk to prepare the campsite. Seemed like this should be a harmless enough experience. I found a spot next to the stream with lots of soft pine needles. Seemed ideal—soft, plus the sound of a gurgling stream to lull me to sleep. However, the monk alerted my travel friend and me that our selection could be dangerous.

"How?" I asked.

The answer was short and clear. "If it rains, you will wake up downstream in another zip code, and instead of a gentle stream gurgle, you will hear the *roar* of the stream."

The reason my proposed campsite was so soft was the settling of the silt and needles from the regular stream flooding over the banks there. It appeared my silence about my camping experience would soon speak for itself. Yes, the truth that I had never camped since being a Cub Scout on an outing in the neighbors' backyard would become all too apparent.

The tent was an old Cub Scout pup tent with all the poles and stakes and so on. There were no instructions, and my friend and I labored hard to get it up correctly. There were frequent episodes of the poles flying apart while we tried to position them in the correct points on the tent.

Taking a break to watch the others erect their tents was not a good idea. Okay, I was back to that feeling of not belonging. I could not believe my eyes. There were two ladies on this outing who simply shook their tent—shook it like I might shake a rug to clean it. *Pop,* they had an instant tent! No poles, just stake it down to the earth. These slender vegan people had somehow intuitively figured this stuff out.

It was warm by now—more so for me after tent pole wrestling. But there were two men who went from long pants and long sleeve shirts to shorts and short sleeves. Yes, and they did not have to run into the tent to change. No. They just unzipped sleeves and pant legs. I noticed others doing this as well. They all seem to live in "white light" blessed worlds. Or I did not get the email about this possibility. How did they know this stuff?

Our evening meal would be an individual job. The monks dubbed it a "mindfulness solitary experience." We were scurrying about the forest floor gathering twigs and bigger branches for the fire for us to heat our dinners. I placed rocks around the firepit to further contain the blaze. I felt like everything was doing just fine. Then while looking about at the other participants fully preparing to receive their knowing nods of approval for our efforts, I realized, *Okay. I am back to not belonging.* File notes for the rest of the trip and future—never raise your head and compare by looking around. In fact, the idea of buying horse blinders seemed good. The two ladies with the instant tent put together an instant stove with these little butane cylinders for fuel. Yes, they flipped open a leather case and screwed together a stove complete with grill top! Where did they find these things?

I felt a bit smug though. Before leaving home to come to the monastery, we'd both buttered two giant potatoes to eat on the trip. They were next wrapped in foil and would be baked in the fire. Well, upon taking the potatoes out of the plastic bag in my pack, it was clear something was wrong. Oh my, they smelled very bad.

The monk came over, and we unwrapped the foil from them. They were black and rancid—apparently the butter and sour cream did not do well after two days in my camping pack. Oh my, that was not good. It also did not bode well for the next night's dinner of a similar item in my sack. I kept it hidden in the sack to avoid further humiliation.

The bag of trail mix we'd put together, also assembled before leaving home, would be our meals for the next forty-eight hours, as my travel friend had done the same thing with his potatoes. My having hidden one of the failed black breads I'd made the day before during kitchen duties meant it would be a big part of tonight's meal. Sorry, they were to be mini loafs but turned out flat.

The beautiful, all-knowing people were at it again. It was the diet. If those potatoes weren't rancid, the meal would have helped me along the vegan diet path—not to mention my sense of confidence.

To add insult to my already injured ego, one of my campfire rocks popped like a mini explosion. Now what? One of the men with the magic clothes explained that the type of rock I'd selected would do that under high heat. I sat dejected. It was not like I'd failed to read or was uneducated—just the opposite. But maybe I wasn't reading topics beyond my comfort zone?

I had not learned these things about camping during my Cub Scout camping training in the neighbors' backyard. Well, it had been thirty years, give or taken, since then—maybe I'd forgotten. I sat rather dejected.

The knowledgeable fellow who explained the rock suggested that we walk together. It was like a nature walk with a lecture. But it wasn't a condescending walk, just very helpful. In fact, it was why I wanted to grow spiritually like him and the other knowledgeable vegetarians—they were always polite and compassionate.

We returned to the campfire area, and I was asked to join them for dinner. I was in training for outdoor cooking, and I figured I could learn just watching him. What he could do with dried food and a canteen of water was simply amazing. He even made chocolate cookies! He tried to explain it was not actual chocolate but a healthy substitute—wish I could remember what it was for future reference.

After evening meditations, I went to sleep. That was not too bad. Everyone else had lots of foodstuff and things like toothpaste tied up in the trees to avoid bear incidents. I took my trail mix and hard flat bread with my tent neighbor's items and hung them from a tree branch.

As an aside, ridding my backpack of all those potatoes lightened my carrying load considerably. My biggest fear that night in the tent was imagining a huge bear slipping from the tree branch where we'd hung our items and crashing through the tent and landing on me. It never happened—thankfully.

The morning was beautiful in the mountains. Or it appeared so through the tent flap. A bathroom was needed, the tent flap was being difficult for us to unzip. I tried to sit up to get a better angle. Well, my arthritis and the damp mountain ground against the tent floor were enough to have my whole body seemingly impossible to bend. This could be serious. Needing to pee in the morning is important for middle-aged men.

Calling out for help was not an option—mainly because of the potential for embarrassment. I tried massaging my back and other parts that were reachable. This worked sort of, but the flap zipper was still an issue. My Swiss Army knife was handy, and the flap was in jeopardy of being slashed.

Fortunately, the monk walked by, simply smiled, and unzipped it for me. And my tent exit was hasty yet made with relative dignity.

After I'd returned from the outdoor privy experience, there was an exercise time for us to limber up for our meditation and sharing session. The limbering up made the meditations work. Breakfast was a generous handful of trail mix and a swig from the canteen. Coffee seemed like a dream state out there to enjoy in the future when we returned to the monastery. Others had these dry packs of coffee. Yes, the same dry food magic with a canteen of water. Should there ever be camping again in the future for me, those tricks would be remembered. At this point, it was a bet I would not wager—that I would ever return to the wild again.

At Camp Granola and here, "sharing" seemed to be a big theme. At first, I would not go beyond "name, rank, and serial number." I let loose with where I lived. That seemed to be okay, which led me to disclose my profession. The monk smiled and reminded me it was not an inquisition but a way for all of us to see ourselves in each other and find ways to support one another.

The next session I did better at personal sharing and found some others had similar notions—it was a strange sensation for me, including both relief and acceptance to experience this time of sharing.

As the week progressed, my ability ranks in outdoorsman ship moved up from the Cub Scout ranks of Bobcat to perhaps Wolf. But the elusive Cub Scout's highest rank of Webelos was clearly not attained. Still, the chance to move forward on this quest was just wonderful. A week with virtually one-to-one dialogue during the canoe paddling was very helpful. If nothing else just the role modeling of nonjudgmental acceptance of me by not only the monks but also the whole group gave me powerful new insights. It was another building block of the new person I was hoping to become. I was starting to see myself becoming like them. This guided my acceptance of those who may not be as aware in areas where I was well versed.

Reinvention of self is not instantaneous. It means being mindful of your inward vision and always working toward that goal. One of the points of confidence that this could work for me had come about years ago. I had failed several times to quit smoking. A very spiritual friend, also a counselor and health PhD student, showed me the way. She helped me put together a vision of myself without cigarettes that was stronger than the current smoking version. Upon my acceptance of that new vision of self, I quit on the Great American Smokeout day and never looked back.

I lamented to her several years after this trip about my dream to be a vegetarian, and an on-the-path, knowing type person. We chatted, but her message was simple. She said, "You know how."

That is when I put together my plan of experiences that would help me achieve the new vision of self. The monastery trip helped, but it was only one of the many adventures that were planned. The difficult part seemed to be my "gift" of making a spectacle of myself and the feelings of not belonging as a result of them.

Oh well. I had a tough hide, and there would be more embarrassing experiences to come. I certainly learned a great deal about Buddhism from the meditations and the teaching sessions where the senior abbot of the monastery would instruct the group. He and the other senior monks were helpful and eager to teach. I did learn that this form of Zen Buddhism might be a bit too rigid for me. Later on my journey, I began a decade of serious study of Vietnamese Buddhism under the brilliant monk Thich Nhat Hanh.

Possible Readings

Suzuki, D. T. *An Introduction to Zen Buddhism.* New York: Grove Press, 1964.

This small book was the first big seller about Buddhism in America. Although D. T. Suzuki wrote at least twelve books, this one, with the introduction by C. G. Jung, was the first exposure to Buddhism for the majority of Americans. The book is basic yet gives all the practical parts of this wonderful philosophy with which we can pursue our lives.

Thich Nhat Hanh. *Living Buddha, Living Christ.* New York: Riverhead Books, 1995.

This national best seller pulls together in an easy reading fashion the points of nexus between Christianity and Buddhism. This book is so moving it feels like the mind and heart of the Buddha are "channeling" through Thich Nhat Hanh.

Kamenetz, Robert. *The Jew in the Lotus.* San Francisco: Harper Collins, 1994.

This book taught me more about the Jewish faith than any popular presswork and helped in my own spiritual journey to understand Jewish mysticism. It bounces the interrelationships of both Buddhism and the Jewish faith in an easy-to-understand fashion.

Schuon, Frithjof. *The Transcendent Unity of Religions.* Wheaton, IL: Theosophical Publishing House, 1993. The reviews refer to this work as treating religion in global terms. Sounds simple, but I recommend you not think of this as an easy, quick read. It is brilliant, and many sections require some degree of time to digest what has been explained. It does not take long to realize this is a very profound book, which takes you on a journey to look at spiritual reality in a whole new framework.

CHAPTER 3

Shopping and Cooking Classes

My early individual attempts at vegetarian cooking at home had gotten off to a tough start. At first it was just eating sans meat. Then I got a cookbook for vegan/ vegetarian use. Well, I had none of the ingredients listed for most of the recipes. To be honest I had never heard of them before. Yes, there were ingredients like, cumin, vinaigrette, and orecchiette. There was a recipes for pistou, which I learned is the French version of Italy's pesto soup. One recipe called for leeks and to use just the pale green and white parts. I had thought leeks were fish.

My attempts had been further complicated by living in a small town, where the food shopping is fine if there are no special needs, like being a vegan. In a small town and not near a metro area, I found none of these ingredients. But learning to shop was another adventure to be shared.

I had been grocery shopping before. And I was considered a good cook by my friends. But this transition to reinvent myself has taken me in directions, places and recipes I'd never visited before in this lifetime.

Here at the entrance to Wegmans, an enormous grocery and specialty food store, the sights and smells were almost overwhelming. The goal this weekend was to shop both Wegmans and Whole Foods, as well as some smaller similar shops. None of these stores were exclusively for vegetarians/vegans. But they did offer a huge selection of options for vegetarians/vegans and also had an extensive selection of organic foods. A close friend who was very knowledgeable in both "vegan" shopping and cooking was my guide for this part of my self-improvement journey.

If you have never been to either of these stores, the sheer magnitude of selection is amazing. For instance, a Wegmans employee explained the store stocks over three hundred cheeses. My lifetime of snacking and eating might cover ten varieties of cheese—if I was allowed to include Velveeta.

The "coach," as my friend would be referred to between us during this trip, quickly cautioned me against any public confession to using Velveeta, except with toasted cheese sandwiches or nacho dips where it is the easiest cheese to melt. I smiled to myself thinking, "*Well, what do you know? The beautiful people do have a pecking order for cheese snobbery.*" That fact alone inched up my sense of belonging. I could proceed with a bit of a smile.

This was not a special or scheduled trip to any of the stores this day, but the coach knew some of the store employees, who gave me a floor plan layout of where items by category were located. This piece of paper was akin to a valuable pirate's treasure map for me. Before the end of our shopping trip, there would be many notes written on it with specific locations—kind of like each *X* marked one of many spots.

We were shopping for ingredients to make pumpkin soup that evening—an easy recipe for me as a person with an eastern European peasant family history. But not so in the organic "veggie" gourmet world. This recipe called for, among other items, fresh lemon grass seasoning. I'd never heard of this seasoning before. All of the stores we visited during this special trip had it available—yes it became an *X* marks the spot for future reference. And, it wasn't just for this ingredient; there were many similar items in the same locale, which were duly noted on my "treasure map."

The remaining items were assembled and we then toured the rest of the store. A scouting trip for me did produce a number of feverishly written location notes. My next trip would be solo, and the need to appear as if shopping here was "second nature" ranked high on my self-esteem index.

Our next trek this day would be to a Whole Foods Market.

We had a similar goal at Whole Foods—to tour, take

notes, and assemble ingredients for a specific recipe. Our recipe was for preparing a vegan cabbage soup. Looking over the recipe caused me to laugh inwardly. It was very similar to one that was a fad diet back in the very late 1990s (around 1996) had called the "cabbage soup diet." I was a professional dieter—or so it seemed-and had tried this diet plan. Over my life, I'd tried just about every best-seller fad diet and could paper my den with diet recipes from the magazines placed next to the grocery checkout line touting the newest "miracle weight-loss" diet plan. Writing an intellectual's guide to dieting book would be a snap.

Of course, this soup would be all fresh and organic items with only a vegetable broth base. The notion of organic has acquired legal presence. Now, to claim a food item is "organic" means there are many hoops to jump through to prove the food item in question is *truly* organic as defined by some local, state, or federal governing body.

For several decades, driving to or from work, I passed various vegetable and fruit stands on the way. One, in particular, was run by an Amish family, with items from their own farm/orchards. Teasing the elderly woman who ran the stand was always light-hearted fun for both of us. During one stop, I offered the observation that she was selling organic foods, to which she quickly replied that her goods should not be called something like that. She told me her family had been raising food the same way for many generations. Duly noted. And I never used the term *organic* with her again.

This family had never used any chemical fertilizers or pesticides on either their farm or orchards. To keep certain pests from the garden, they planted flowers like zinnias, among others that are very good for keeping pests away from the plants naturally. Her family utilized "ley lines" of the earth's natural forces and power to aid in the growth as well.

Now, many dispute the "new age" notion of such things—but this Amish family was hardly new age, and they really didn't care about the intellectual debate. For them, the generations of results spoke for themselves. Their produce was of excellent quality, and that was always good enough for me. That said, this was my singular Amish experience, so I cannot testify that this activity as the norm for all Amish.

So, back to the shopping trip. Like Wegmans, Whole Foods market was impressive. Not just a place to buy groceries, it is enjoyable to have a good cup of coffee to drink while shopping, and the cup holder on the shopping cart is a nice plus. I also liked the little sample snacks from the vendors. But the best part was catching a vision of the pub inside the store, where I could get a nice cold IPA from some microbrewery!

This IPA beer craze was new for me. Back when I was a twentysomething, if someone had a case of Michelob or Coors, for example, it was as good as a person could ever want. It was taking time for me to develop a taste for the "hoppy" beers that seemed to be all the rage with many local microbreweries. For my taste, they all seemed so bitter. But my beautiful "veggie" friends all drink it, so it seemed to be part of the mandatory learning curve to "to get there."

My friend and shopping coach was great at weaving us through the store, explaining how to pick out fresh herbs and spices, describing what constitutes a good deal, and identifying acceptable substitutes if the items I wanted were too high-priced.

The only real trauma at this point was my sniffing the various herbs and spices too vigorously. Some went into my lungs, which triggered a violent asthma attack, along with the stark realization of not being able to get a breath. It was scary for everyone around us, as well as myself.

People were screaming, "Dial 9-1-1," "Call an ambulance!" or, "Is there a doctor in the store?"

Well, a puff or two of my inhaler and some water from an off-duty nurse, and all was well again. Sitting on the floor, leaning against a counter, my mind tried to make sense out of the all the troubles that continued to befall me in this endeavor to be on the path to self-improvement. Could someone like me just be jinxed? Lots of people were sniffing things in the store, and they did not end up sitting on the floor.

My friend believed it was a case of trying too hard, like sniffing too deeply and vigorously. Good grief—I might even have to pace my sniffing when we got home to learn to cook all this stuff.

The ride home was full of chatter about what we'd both experienced during our shopping for these ingredients. It would be great to be led through the preparation process by an accomplished vegetarian cook. My guess was that it would be like the advantage one has by starting to learn to play golf—or any individual sport for that matter—by taking lessons up front. It avoided unlearning bad habits.

I had taken cooking classes before. These were typically with twenty to thirty others at a beach resort to learn how to cook seafood. I love the ambiance of the beach more than actually sitting on the sand and just staring at waves continually lapping into shore. Maybe it was because of the fact that, no matter how thickly sunscreen lotion was applied, a sunburn would appear on some part of my exposed body—meaning, after about an hour on the beach, it would be time for me to find something else to do.

Stay with me here. We'll get back to vegetarian cooking in a moment. So, up and down the East Coast, I have library cards—yes, library cards. It amuses my friends that someone would go the beach and end up in a library. Well, the libraries at Hilton Head, South Carolina, and Lewes, Delaware, to name just two, are places where I have spent a great deal of time. Both boast interesting lecture series, art shows, and daily copies of the *Times* to read, plus a great selection of books available to check out. But the most fun are the classes. These libraries have sessions on about every topic imaginable. I also take full advantage of hands-on cooking classes offered at several of the more upscale restaurants at both beach towns.

My first lesson at a gourmet seafood restaurant

kitchen in Lewes resulted in a problem. We were being taught how to slice and filet fish. Seemed harmless enough, and the instructor did warn us how very sharp the knives were. True to form, just when it seemed like the skill set was coming my way, a slip of the knife occurred and resulted in a quick trip to urgent care for stiches. Tip to carving novices—do not look up and smugly smile to classmates, as the speed of a very sharp knife through fish is rapid, and one's skin can be filleted as easily as a fish skin.

Enough of war stories—you get the point. As an aside, for just a few dollars more, you can request the shop to cut and skin your fish as the recipe dictates. It saves time, as well as some stitches and a trip to urgent care.

Back to veggie cooking. At my kitchen, with all the ingredients out, the coach began with what will be a very methodical teaching method. As mentioned earlier, I am an overall good cook. My kitchen is fairly well organized from the pots and pans to the run of the mill spices and cooking utensils.

My first real training in being a cook came in college when, after being badly injured as a football player, I found myself in need of a job and the immediate necessity to actually study. I landed a job in a gourmet Spanish restaurant. Over the course of my employment there, I became a knowledgeable cook in this genre and, over time, expanded my repertoire. But the expansions were never into vegan/vegetarian cooking.

The coach's methodical approach to teaching this

genre of food worked well for me and tended not to omit any points along the way. It was like an epiphany during the lecture. I had been approaching vegetarian cooking all wrong. It had been my protocol to cook what was in my normal eating patterns, simply leaving out the meat; chicken; and, with great pain, even fish. But that was so far off the mark.

For most of my life, making soup had been rather straightforward. I either opened several cans of premade soup or used various broth bases available in the grocery store and sometimes just added water to a dry mix. I felt special if the can label disclosed it was organic soup.

Well, both the pumpkin soup and the cabbage soup were a big new experience. Pans all over the stove were sautéing ingredients; there was endless chopping of others. I had never really cut up a fresh pumpkin before. I just usually opened a can of pumpkin. Well, I did cut a pumpkin for Halloween once, but it was not to eat—just to carve an off-center face to scare little kids with a candle inside. Only the neighbor's cat was ever frightened by it.

The coach showed me how to prepare the seeds for later roasting and use as a healthy snack. Apparently, there are several seeds like this I have been wasting my whole life. I grow sunflowers in the garden for artistic reasons; this year, I will harvest some to eat. The plus side is saving money, as I regularly buy both dried varieties to use with my meals. One of my friends asked if I was turning into a self-sufficient survivalist. Good grief, it's just cooking a few kinds of seeds! I do use the seeds and walnuts with my morning yogurt or oatmeal. Besides, the combo adds flavor to both yogurt and oatmeal, and it is a healthy combination to eat.

Good vegetarian cooking is very multidimensional. I was learning that it's also about presentation of the meal—how the spices create the great appetizing scents, as well as the artistry of the craft of cooking. To my surprise, it involved, by necessity, balancing of enzymes, proteins, and carbs. This notion had great appeal to my intellectual side.

The coach did recommend a good nutritionist as a reference person. There are some who, while good, are not vegans and tend to stick only with the traditional food pyramid, where meat and dairy are the king and queen of healthy eating. The coach had names of two vegan PhDs to contact on the subject of vegan nutrition. That was good advice and could provide help in avoiding health issues by not properly balancing the diet. Leaving out dairy and meat complicate the task of getting the required daily amounts of necessary nutrients in the diet.

There was a study published in 2015 by the national Academy of Science. The study highly touted a vegan diet and how it protected against such things as hypertension and type-2 diabetes; reduced cardiovascular disease risks; and reduced obesity, with all its accompanying negative health issues. The diet seemed to rest on the vegan eating regimen being low in saturated fats, among other health benefits.

The experts did caution that some nutritional areas

are more difficult to achieve in the vegan plan. For example, it is cited that achieving the daily nutritional levels for calcium, omega-3 fatty acids, and vitamin B12 is harder with the vegan regimen.

Yet in 2016, the United Nations declared that year as the "International Year of Pulses" to heighten awareness of healthy, sustainable food options. It is true that animal products offer a "one-stop shop" for all the essential amino acids the body requires. But the recommended pulses include dried peas, kidney beans, chickpeas, fava beans, and black beans, to name a few, which can also provide the body's amino acid needs. But the experts there cautioned that this pulses approach needs regular planning and focus to combine the correct grains with the beans and so on to achieve the equal results of animal products. They further caution that these foods are high in roughage and can result in bloating and some quick trips to the toilets, as I can personally attest to.

What surfaces as a key trigger for my staying on this path to self-improvement is the reinforcement that being a vegetarian cook will provide a way to strengthen the "new image" of myself that is so necessary for this change to stick. Over the years, it seems every self-help philosophy fad book had found its way into my hands. But nothing was sustained for any real length of time, much like the many diets in my life. This vision of myself as a vegetarian may work if only I can stop cutting myself, snorting spices into my lungs, or disrupting spiritual events with cramps or diarrhea.

The cliché is that every journey begins with a first step; let's hope my second or third steps stop being so eventful and filled with negativity. It is important for me personally to achieve this goal.

But like any project, it seems to continue to grow in magnitude. It's sort of like a "simple" home repair, where each step requires more presteps, or halfway in, I realize there are various things going wrong that must be done or my simple repair will not work. I am now journaling even more carefully to be sure I don't forget steps like consulting a nutritionist. However, it was quickly pointed out that any nutritionist would promote the eating hierarchy triangle, and I needed to be ready to discuss how I wanted to eat beyond being "vegetatian-ish."

A quick look at popular eating plans offered the notable best-selling names—ketogenic diet, military diet, Paleo diet, Intermittent Fasting Diet, the Mediterranean diet, Mind Diet, and the WW diet. There were even plans that suggest we eat according to our body type.

There was a relatively new book out about body type eating by Phil Catudal and Stacey Colino, *Just Your Type: The Ultimate Guide to Eating and Training Right for Your Body Type."* This book and others in the body type genre divide all of us into three types according to our body type—ectomorph, mesomorph, and endomorph. Ectomorphs are long, thin, lanky people who have trouble gaining weight—obviously not my body type. It is suggested that people in this group divide their intake of carbs, proteins, and fats along 45-35-20 percent line, which is lower in protein and fat, with higher carbs. A ketogenic diet will never work in theory for this group.

The second category is mesomorph people—those who have the perfect hourglass figures with nice muscle tone. Their caloric intake is evenly divided along the three categories.

The last category is endomorphs, who have more body fat. The polite term here is *stocky men*. Take a wild guess which I am. Endomorphs recommended carb, protein, and fat division is a bell curve—with a 20-40-20 per cent distribution.

The theory of this type of eating plan is to help the follower avoid fad diets, which may not work or even be counterproductive. As suspected, there is a host of other experts who dispute the science behind the body type theory of eating.

As will be discussed in more detail about my own plan choice, it will not to be along any particular notion or theory. It is to be a part of a larger life reinvention where eating fits into the overall larger scheme.

Okay. It's time to look at the plan and see if I have neglected looking at any specific area. It turns out there is one? It's one that's implied but not yet addressed—exercise.

Yes, exercise. About every diet I ever tried always mentioned "proper exercise" as part of the successful plan. Some went on explaining at greater lengths, and others gave not much more than the two words—*proper exercise.* Yet, it is a necessary piece of the self-puzzle reinvention for my success. I decided to obtain the help of a professional in the design of this phase. I did not plan to have an exercise coach accompany me to carry out the exercise visits, just the design.

Some Readings

If what you're looking for is a cookbook, then just about every weight-loss book has countless numbers of recipes included usually at the back part of the book. There are great magazines, like *Vegetation Times*, with helpful articles and recipes as well.

Caldwell, B. Esselstyn Jr., *Prevent and Reverse Heart Disease.* New York: Avery, 2007.
  I received this book at a program in my hometown area, where two very informed and energetic ladies lead a program of healthy eating based on a plant-based diet. Besides the helpful recipes it has a compelling argument for how we can abolish heart disease by changing our diet. It is a plant-based and oil-free program of eating with many sound results.

Hunt, Sally, PhD. *365 Easy Vegetarian Recipes.* Cookbook Resources, 2011.
  In addition to many individual recipes cut out of magazines this is the only dedicated recipe book on my shelf. Meaning, it is not part of some proposed eating plan-just as the title offers they are short and

easy to make meals. Too many esoteric ingredients often rule out for me trying a specific recipe.

Drucker, Ronald P. *The Code of Life*, 2012.
I am a believer in the notion that, given the correct care and feeding, the human body can heal many of its own woes. The argument presented in this book is that our cells are designed to do just that—yes, to rejuvenate and heal themselves. It is a good read, which also teaches the reader the science behind the cellular healing process.

Catudal, Phil, and Stacey Colino. *Just Your Type: The Ultimate Guide to Eating for Your Body Type*. New York: Da Capo Books, 2019.

The above book was referred to in this chapter.

D'Adamo, Peter J. *Eat Right 4 Your Type*. New York: Berkley Books, 2016.

This book was an early best seller in the body type eating genera of diets.

CHAPTER 4

Trip to a Health Club

"Okay. It's time!" a friend of mine proclaimed.

It was time to join a "health club." I'd been consumed by self-talk about this for much of my life. There were many arguments in my head for why I should join. It wasn't like there was never a membership card in my wallet. Yes, I would join some club and then never or rarely go, yet pay faithfully till the contract expired. On the other hand, I'd been a faithful member of the local YMCA dating back to my teenage years. I looked at my friend with the unspoken question—why this "joining" would be any different.

As we'd been friends for decades, he read my mind and said he could recommend someone to help with this process.

I had a veritable health club of exercise machines in the basement. Many were just like new—meaning rarely used! Visitors to this area of my home probably see infomercials pass before their eyes as they tour the room. All are reminders of my annual pledge to lose weight and regain the "old" body form of yesteryear. In the garage, my bike proudly hangs on the wall. Truth be told, it needs the tires reinflated just about every time it's taken from the wall rack for me to ride.

No doubt, an expert was needed this time if I was to succeed at a consistent plan of exercising. Of course, the beautiful vegetarian people, who I so wanted to be like, probably needed no such help. In my mind, they were, from birth, imbued with exercise ability and desire deep in their DNA. But I was convinced I could change and improve on this journey. Vegetarianism was a good umbrella theme for the journey, as it encompassed many needed steps to grow on the path of self-improvement.

Now, in my defense, I golfed, hiked, and had played squash when the back was more amenable to that sport. So, I was never a classic couch potato.

What made this venture different was the intent. The intention was to create a program of targeted exercises to promote my flexibility, balance, and muscle tone and enhance the cardio system on some regular basis. Especially, as the middle-aged years passed on by, a well-designed routine of exercise would promote a healthier lifestyle long into the future retirement years. So, the need was to now find someone who could provide this assistance.

No doubt, there were many ways to find such a person. Options ranged from local hospitals, which promote a healthy lifestyle, to exercise and fitness coaches. My local hospital in Chambersburg has such a facility, which is staffed with true experts. Of course the local YMCA has similar help, as do other health clubs in about every community. Do go on line and check credentials of the people who arrive on your own final list to choose from.

My expert turned out to be a lady personal trainer by trade, and she brought a friend. The young man, her friend, had worked in one of the local health clubs for years and had recently gone into business for himself. Both were very personable and easy to talk with. Of course, both were vegans, perfect bodies, the whole works. That part was hard. Why couldn't there be a less-than-perfect-bodied trainer/helper? I had to confess to them that, considering what I needed to do to come in the *vicinity* of them physically and eating-wise, I might as well just go have a chili dog and a beer, followed up with a nap.

To their credit, this comment did not phase them. The process began with lots of questions about me and my dreams in terms of what I looked forward to happening as a result of joining a club. That did resonate with what I'd learned so far on my path. Here again was the notion of me maintaining that positive picture of self—the new and reinvented me. Positive self-talk and imaging is so critical in all phases of self-improvement and more so in the beginning, till some results are visible. This vision, combined with self-recognition of my personality, could help narrow down the club options—yes, club options. Even in my smallish town where I live, there are many possibilities.

There was one difficult issue that needed to be revealed to the duo helping me. Despite how hard the exercise routine at any gym or health club in the past, my weight went up with exercise. The duo wasn't phased and simply responded that overeating the calorie burn at the gym would always result in weight gain. The key was to carefully plan the eating so that, after a workout when the hunger struck, lots of vegetables were the option to satisfy the emerging hunger pains.

Health clubs do vary. I know many seem to have similar equipment and locker rooms. But when you step back and compare, each does have a personality or a theme it supports. I made a list of all the items for comparison purposes and even took the opportunity for short trial visits. My experts highly suggested this and told me to ask for a trial plan if this option wasn't visibly advertised. All the clubs I asked were glad to do that.

Some were very large clubs, which could accommodate hundreds of patrons at a time if necessary. That meant the equipment I wanted was usually available without me waiting. And these large clubs were usually the lower price per month.

Some others were expensive and very fancy, right down to teak wood lockers. The expensive facilities usually had lots of staff to help and coach you during the workouts, with pep talks to help achieve your plan that was written out on paper; they tended to be smaller and less crowded.

Others were part of a larger mission-based organization like a YMCA or YWCA, where the health club was but one item on their menu of activities.

Still others were very small, with a highly defined offering. For example, there were circuit-training clubs, where you would come in and perform a defined workout for thirty minutes, moving from machine to machine in a preset timing sequence. The option to just show up and do what you wished was certainly available. This is not to imply these programs aren't successful—for those who follow the defined circuit protocol these patrons do see success. The kind of regimentation in circuit training sort of appealed to me—in that it took away thinking, and I could fit the workout into a routine. However, in my hometown, the circuit-training clubs were dominated by women members, and I had to assess my comfort at being the only male on the circuit at any given time.

Some health clubs specialized in a particular exercise or sport, like racquet clubs where the workout options were handball, squash, racket ball, tennis, or pickle ball. All these were a great cardio workout but tended to offer less on the machines or free weights. I found that, if I wanted both racket sports with health club facilities and maybe even the option to swim laps, then a multimission place like a YMCA had it all.

See what I mean by personality? The choices and combinations were many, and all had some appeal. It came down to being specific about my targets for what I wanted to achieve in developing my physical body. My expert coach lady was good at steering my thinking to the specifics. And being specific would save me some money by not buying more than I would use right now. She was correct. When I achieve this targeted goal, I could always set new goals, which might involve changing my health club. It wasn't a lifetime commitment to any one club.

I must admit to being relieved at making the choice. I also took her up on an offer to help me set my goals and the plan of successive activities with a reasonable time frame to get there. Never in my life to date had I ever gone to a health club with any sort of plan in mind, let alone on paper. I would just show up and hope to get sweaty and tired, take a shower, and leave.

So, my first trip to the chosen club by myself—plan in hand—as I was walking in the door, I was nervous. It wasn't as bad as expected. That feeling I always seemed to have about not fitting in places was there, but it wasn't so overwhelming now. I had visited here and met the staff, and I was familiar with the machines and layout. The positive self-talk was helping. No wandering around nervous. I knew what sequence my visits would take. There must be something to this planning.

I was on an elliptical machine—"how did they tell me to enter my weight?" "Good grief, there were a lot of buttons." I couldn't wait for artificial intelligence to get to health clubs. I could enter all my stuff once, and it would auto appear as soon I entered my personal code. "Quit dreaming." I figured out the buttons. Now to just enjoy myself.

Wow, this felt like another piece of that 360-degree puzzle of growth just might be in place for me to get to my ultimate goal. Yes, I would be among the vegetarian, fit, aware, and beautiful people.

So, now I knew how to shop, I was getting the eating part, and I did tai chi and yoga. And I was doing a workout in peace and enjoying the people I was meeting. I read a lot of research about being physically fit and being at a good weight level. It appeared, according to the studies, that the best way any person could hold down his or her own health care cost was to not be ill in the first place. Eating right and being fit won that game, aside from accidents and catastrophic illnesses beyond my control. And, the cost of a health club was a fraction of the cost of a hospital visit or a lot of prescription medications. The experts claimed a regular health management plan could possibly make many of the prescriptions just go away as unnecessary.

So, it was time for me to look at the list of things I may need to learn or do to keep moving on this path. Spiritual growth, perhaps in Buddhism, beyond just the meditation that I was practicing now was on the list. And a recurrent theme in all my lessons and visits was developing a sense of positive self-awareness. Neither of these appeared to be areas where I would encounter self-harm or embarrass myself. But again, who would have believed a trip to a supermarket could have turned out with me on the floor on the verge of blacking out from the inability to catch my breath? So the journey to reinvent myself continued.

A Look at Nutrition

One of the most humorous conversations experienced on this path to reinvention of self-occurred with a friend who was knowledgeable on nutrition. She was counseling me about conscious food choices, as well as conscious quantity limits at the same time. The flow of the dialogue shifted to methods of self-reward when I achieved incremental "wins." She asked what the positive reinforcements were that would present the most meaning to me.

This sort of reward system was something not associated with my past. I would set highly specific goals and either hit them with a smile or go into self-loathing when they were missed. My response resulted in her eyes slightly widening, a smirk on her upturned lips and lots of eye blinks.

The answer was not meant to be glib, and my vocal tone was straightforward when answering her—"low golf score, lots of opportunities for lovemaking, and driving too fast in my old Porsche on a country road."

She leaned toward me and said there needed to be a rethinking of my life positions on personal growth, as the rewards just mentioned were not particularly useful for sustained behavior change. Her answer was true and set out a rigorous pace of reading self-help books recommended by friends and others. It also crystallized the notion of this journey being much more than weight loss.

When looking back on the many decades of my

focus on weight loss, one point became clear—the plans had all worked. Just about all of them were what I'd call elimination eating programs.

What does this "elimination" program mean? In the most basic definition, as explained to me by a nutritionist, it's that everything we eat is in one of three broad nutrient categories. These are proteins, fats, or carbohydrates. That said, fruits are a tricky carbohydrate, for example. Despite the halo effect surrounding fruit, they can be sources of significant carbohydrates but mostly in terms of simple sugars, glucose and fructose—hence, it's not allowed in high-protein, low- or no-carb diets. But many low-carb vegetables are on the "okay" low-carb diet regimen. Carbs like pasta and breads are much higher in carbs than fruits. See, it's tricky.

Back to elimination eating. As I was taught by my nutritional advisor (who I then fact-checked), if you actually eliminate any one of the three, you will, by simple chemistry, lose weight. Again, the high-protein, high-fat diets eliminate carbohydrates. Back in 1972, the famous *Dr. Atkins' New Diet Revolution* was published and ushered in the era of elimination diet research and, of course, many copycat high-protein diets.

Of course, I immediately bought a copy of the book and became a disciple of the notion. I was living in New York City working for a major Wall Street firm at that point in time. I was new to Wall Street, and the money was scarce during the initial career years. This diet became easy to follow in a strange way. My roommate and I decided to go on the diet and soon learned that canned tuna was very cheap and a relatively new soda, diet Fresca, was even less expensive. It was the perfect Atkins diet of forced choice eating due to our lack of funds. We went early to work, as our firm offered free scrambled eggs, toast, and coffee for the early birds. We did not eat the toast. It helped our psyche to say when asked about our new eating habits that we were part of the new "Atkins revolution" rather than admit we were too poor to eat better. The weight loss was rapid and noticeable.

I could clearly remember the almost devotional allegiance we both had to the daily peeing on a ketone test strip. How happy or sad we were, as well as our outlook for the day, became dependent on how dark purple the test strip turned. The darker the purple, the more we were in ketosis, and consequently, the faster the weight came off. The high-fat nature of this eating protocol meant you felt fuller—you were virtually never hungry, despite eating less with corresponding fewer calories.

Here is a short explanation why this works. The body becomes a fat-burning furnace. The state of ketosis we so highly coveted is a metabolic process where the body uses up glycogen stores for energy when carbohydrates are not readily available. This occurs by breaking down the body's stored fat into fatty acids. These fatty acids are changed into ketones, which now become the new or alternate fuel source for the body. Many of you reading this may already be familiar with this, and there is a large body of literature that can take you into the complex aspects of the process if that is needed in your psyche.

When fact-checking myself in this writing I came across twelve ketogenic diet blogs. The lure to join this diet fad read to the effect of asking the reader if he or she wanted a low-carb, high-fat eating fest diet program with a quick weight-loss reward. It made me smile.

As an aside, there are also risks associated with ketogenic eating plans. The nature of the food consumed is higher in cholesterol, which can increase blood level cholesterol associated with heart disease. Secondly, ketogenic diets show calcium is lost in the urine. This may lead to decreases in bone density and a higher risk of osteoporosis.

Whether it is this or any other diet, do consult your physician, especially if there are current health issues or concerns. Yes, this is my required warning with this type of writing.

However, as time went on and income rose modestly, along came tastier food choices, and our weight loss quickly reversed.

Later in time, I tried the diet that just eliminated fats. Similar story to the high-protein experiment. Rapid weight loss was followed by rapid regain, as the eating regimen varied to include even the simplest fats like butter on toast and cream for coffee.

It was clear that a 360-degree look at eating needed to be adopted for any successful long-term weight loss. It needed to be a lifestyle change. To yo-yo up and down in body weight is also a potentially dangerous health issue.

I did not wish to have a nutritionist who would simply pull out and dust off the food pyramid, with meat and dairy at the pinnacle of the food chain and vegetables and grains at the bottom. So it took some work. But the simplest way I found to thin the field of possible candidates was to ask for references and speak to them. I was not listening for personality issues as much as listening for creativity and willingness to look at vegetarian alternatives, with instruction on how to balance the necessary enzymes for positive good health.

When I conducted my own research to be ready for the nutritionist, it became apparent that nutritionists are not all of one mind on what constitutes a balanced ratio among fats, proteins, and carbohydrates. I am also an economist among my various professional training genres. No two economists can agree on anything, so the variance among nutritionists did not become a cause for alarm. Various experts put the ratios at one of these:

- 40 percent carbs, 30 percent proteins, 30 percent fats
- 45–65 percent carbs, 10–35 percent proteins, 20–35 percent fats

As you can see, there's a lot of room for argument. My goal was to find one or two to be open to the notion of vegetarian eating in a healthy, balanced manner.

In today's world of protein being available through

pea protein isolates, it is much safer for men than the earlier era of only eating soy proteins. Yes, for men, too much soy ingestion is a long-term problem, especially with advanced prostate health issues. If the prostate issue has not spread beyond advanced, the long-term influence is not as significant and possibly only minor. Well, just the idea it could be an issue at some point was enough for me to avoid soy and as many other isoflavones as possible. Besides these facts, at Camp Granola, I'd learned the gaseous effect of eating too much soy and had no desire to go through that again.

Well, my first try at vegetarian eating had been decades ago and very difficult, as soy was a relative newcomer and the pea protein isolates were nowhere to be found. An overabundance of high fiber beans came with its own serious issues—like being caught on a subway with no easy fast exit for a men's room.

However, in the diet/fitness world, things get trendy in a hurry. So putting together the ideal combination of proteins, fats, and carbohydrates in today's world has rapidly evolved into formulas for people like me to craft our own individual macronutrient ratio. This ratio is simply computing the optimum combination of fats, proteins, and carbs.

Do not get nervous about what is coming next, as there is no lack of articles and social media assistance on how to compute this. Many offer some form of macronutrient calculator. Most recently, the dialogue in the fitness centers—as many are called rather than gyms or health clubs—includes the term *macros* in conversations about fitness goals. The American College of Lifestyle Medicine believes that none of us "dreamers" who are hoping to become one of the beautiful people will get there without due attention to our individual macros.

As a retired professor, I expected that various universities would enter this research arena. Washington State University, among others, define macros as the effective grouping of the three nutrient groups of fats, proteins, and carbohydrates, which my body will require to become one of the beautiful people—or to at the least be in a sustainably successful eating protocol. The generally accepted breakdown of fuel equivalents of each category are:

- One gram of protein = four calories
- One gram of fat = nine calories
- One gram of carbohydrates = four calories

From all this, an expected acronym did emerge. IIFYM or "if it fits your macro diet." What appeals enough for me to pay attention to all this is the confirmed wonderful reality of the research that no single eating regimen fits everyone? It recognizes individual differences. These differences include personal characteristics, daily living activities, and one's personal visions and goals. The approach is numbers driven, and this fact alone may put some people off. But it is not difficult, and even if I or others choose not to go to this depth, the understanding of why the individual differences are key factors will still direct the effort and keep it on the correct path.

It involves three steps with some work within each step. Broadly, the three are

- figure my basal metabolic rate (BMR);
- add up my Total Daily Energy Output (TDEO); and
- Finally, pin down my personal calorie surplus or deficit.

The way I was taught to compute the BMR is based on the Harris-Benedict formula:

- BMR for women: $65 + (4.35 \times \text{weight}) + (4.71 \times \text{height in inches}) - (4.71 \times \text{age})$
- BMR for men: $66 + (6.23 \times \text{weight}) + (12.7 \times \text{height in inches}) - (6.8 \times \text{age})$

I do not know how the Harris-Benedict research team came up with all these factors. They are, and have been, well accepted in this field, so their factors are good enough for me to accept them as valid.

Counting TDEO does, in a minor way, take into account daily living activity levels:

- Modest levels means 1–3 days of workouts. Therefore, BMR $\times$ 1.375 = number of calories to consume.

- Active levels range means 5–7 days of workouts. BMR × 1.725 = number of calories to consume.

The final part is relatively easy. For me, it means having a clear vision of self that I wish to maintain in the new lifestyle—that is, in simple terms, to maintain, lose, or gain weight.

If the wish is to simply maintain the current weight, the input and output must be equal. To lose weight, I need to have a deficit of calories of between 15 to 25 percent less than TDEO. As confessed earlier, I have been in excess of TDEO because of basic hunger after a big workout. I have no interest in gaining muscle weight—another option here. But the surplus over TDEO should be in favor of proteins, or the result will not be lean muscle mass weight gain but simple body fat gains in weight.

This is all I really need for the basic macro management tracking. However, I have met others in the health club who go beyond this basic tracking to indexes and algorithms that vary with the type of exercise chosen. For the readers interested in this, just Google *macros*, and there are articles that will take you to these calculations.

When doing the above calculations myself, the BMR = 2,000. Next, I needed to find my daily TDOE, which multiplied the BMR × 1.375 = 2,750. Yes, I am a modest category workout person. Three days are at the gym, plus two golfing (golf is not a heavy workout).

Hence, the lower multiplication figure with BMR to get my total daily energy output number.

Now, in order to lose weight, I had to come up with a daily eating calorie deficit between 15 to 25 percent. I chose a goal of a 25 percent daily deficit. Next, I had to multiply my TDOE by 75 percent to get my daily deficit calorie eating number—2,750 × .75 = 2,062.

I knew my personality and knew I wouldn't walk the aisles of a grocery store with a calculator in hand figuring my TDOE numbers before buying food. But, I would have some prefigured numbers of items I planned to regularly consume. And from these, I would then prepare the meals accordingly—meaning my numbers would not be precise but within the ballpark. Hence, I chose the larger 25 percent deficit number to give me a cushion. But the need for expert guidance and instruction was desired in this initial phase.

A closely related anachronism to BMR is BMI. BMI stands for body mass index. The typical way it is calculated is a height-weight ratio and is not necessarily very useful. This simple BMI makes too many assumptions about the "sameness" of everyone involved. There are more sophisticated measurements. I do suggest going to the CDC's website and taking advantage of its BMI calculator for an easier way to handle this.

A notch up on the sophistication level is the Smart Body Mass Index (SBMI). The SBMI has the same height/weight information but includes age and sex as well. There is a fun website that is SBMI based and, also includes information on ethnicity and diet information, thus giving a more accurate reading. At the end of the chapter, there is a link to this site. Please do fill out the quick and easy questionnaire for a free analysis.

Another notch up on BMI analysis uses waist measurements, under the premise that body fat carried at our midsection is more dangerous than that carried on our hips and thighs. There are also BMI calculations that include a comparison of wrist circumference to that of the waist circumference to gain even more refinement.

Why all the trouble to gain more sophistication here? Basic BMI calculations are not very accurate for assessing an optimum weight in certain groups. For example, some ethnic groups, like South Asians, Chinese, and Japanese populations, show less than optimum findings for the basic BMI measure and must use more sophisticated calculators. For those in the category of serious workout athletes, it's not very accurate. The same is true for groups like bodybuilders, weight lifters, and high-performance-type athletes; pregnant women; older folks; people with eating disorders or issues; and those with physical disabilities, to name a few.

The basic BMI was always an issue for me, as I was a linebacker and boxer in my younger years, which involved weight training. At the peak of those years, the basic BMI showed myself and many of the football players as overweight and at moderate health risk. Again, at the end of this chapter is a second link to another website that includes waist in the calculations. For the most part, I simply keep my own BMI as a footnote to my medications/vitamin chart, for use when visiting my health care providers to counter their inadequate BMI numbers.

All these calculations for BMR and BMI have their linkage to our nutritional choices.

So, my search for a nutritionist did take some time but I managed to find several persons who became very helpful. Staying with one expert was preferred, but professionals do tend to move about. My search did lead me to the macros argument as well. My guess was that it would involve me getting some basic rules of thumb to follow in eating, as well as several workout protocols that matched with them. For example, it was suggested that I engage in interval training to reduce belly fat. This would not be a daily activity, but I had to have some idea of the max TDEO as not to outeat my calorie burn, both on the active gym days and the lesser golf days.

The lack of discussion about vitamins is not an oversight. There is no lack of published material about taking supplements. Along with the material is a lot of confusing data that seems to contradict itself. Meaning, one well-respected journal will positively support the use of vitamin supplements, while another will say just the opposite. Again, always consult your medical provider before starting a new program of supplements, especially if you are on prescription medications as there may be drug interaction issues.

Personally, supplements are used in my scheme of nutrition as targeted items. Meaning, they are selected to help with a specific health issue. For example, I have a lot of osteoarthritis, and the pharmaceuticals are said to be hard on the kidneys and liver. Of course, as the kidneys go, so goes the heart—eventually. So, I use fish oil and turmeric. Turmeric is a spice, but it's a "wonder spice" that reduces inflammation. The combined targeted result is no over the counter or prescription drugs are necessary for handling my arthritis.

My awareness here is, if vitamin/herb supplements are to be in your nutrition mix, then research well and pick certified / well-tested brands. My source for third party certification/testing is from—drum roll please—Dr. Oz. He listed Consumer Lab, NSF International, and USP on his show. The web addresses for these sources are at the end of this chapter in the added readings section. This is not meant to be a negative to the great work by Dr. Oz I obviously watched it to acquire this information. His programs focusing on health have brought under the umbrella of awareness countless numbers of citizens who did not have this knowledge prior to their becoming fans of Dr. Oz.

In looking over my areas of concentration there is one area mentioned but included little in the way of actual design or research so far The spiritual component. If this 360-degree reinvention of self is to happen, then the spiritual ingredient must be a vital part. This will be my next area of focus.

Websites and Suggested Reading

The link for the Smart BMI
Smartbmicalculator.com

The link for the BMI calculator including waist
Healthdirect.gov.au/body-mass-index-bmi-and-waist-
circumference.

Atkins, Robert C, MD. *Dr. Atkins' New Diet Revolution*,
Evans & Company. First published 1972, several
revisions since.

This book started the popular high-protein craze.
There is a host of supporting books now that vary
from recipes to carb counters. Dr. Atkins clearly
explains the science behind his arguments for the
low-carb approach.

https://www.healthline.com/health/too-much-protein

For those wishing to examine the arguments for
caution in using one of the many variants of high-
protein diets, go to this link. It is well done and
concise.

Here are the links from Dr. Oz.
- Consumer Lab—consumerlab.com
- NSF International—NSF.org
- USP—usp.org

Endicott, Lanny. *Compassion Fatigue, Burnout & Stress.* Oral Roberts University Press.

This final reading option may appear out of place, as it is not traditional exercise or nutrition oriented. But as an active consultant in the medical / health care field, I often encountered employees who resisted fitness programs. They argued they were just absolutely in a chronic state of fatigue. General overall health not being an issue for them, it was my awareness that many suffered from compassion fatigue. Endicott's book describes compassion fatigue, burnout, and stress. It offers self-assessment tools. It also goes into the spiritual aspect of compassion fatigue, with ideas and suggestions.

CHAPTER 5

The Spiritual Ingredient

The idea of a spiritual component included in the goal to become one of the beautiful people was first touched upon in the discussion with the trip to the Zen monastery. This spiritual aspect has not been absent in my life. I just never connected it to weight loss, fitness, and overall health. The discussion now will go deeper into spirituality and even argue," Why add this?"

The truly beautiful people I wished to emulate were not defined solely by their physical appearance. True, losing weight and having a more fit appearance was important. But the broader definition of beautiful people on the wish list to hopefully emulate were those who seemed to have a special quality that could be associated with an inner spiritual direction in their lives. My self-vision was not to be a clone of an anorexic model with only a nice exterior beauty.

Let's begin by clarifying some basic differences between religion and spiritual direction.

Many years ago, the difference between religion and spirituality was brought home to me in a most unusual setting. This is not to say there is not a fine line in the difference between the two. But when I was a doctoral student, a law professor pointed out the difference as clearly as has ever been presented. His explanation started with the notion that the root of religion is the dogma of each faith. It's agreed upon and set beliefs, practices, and articles, which dictate how each member will conduct him or herself. This indicates that religion is shared by a community or group. Most certainly, it typically involves a relationship to a divine entity or God. The term *theology*, as translated from the ancient original language, simply means "God talk" and, thus, is more readily associated with formal religious activities and study.

Spirituality is somewhat different. It is more of an individual practice and has as its primary area of concern seeking inner peace and life purpose. The experts offer that it frequently focuses on transcendent questions and may have a relationship to a superior being or force (like nature). It is not uncommon to see an existential perspective on life, death, and the reality of life and the world.

Religion often tends to be a more objective experience. To support the objectivity, there are buildings—the church buildings, for example—and agreed upon books of scripture. Religion has lots of rituals and rites—marriage and baptism are just two. There seem to be lots of observances. Hinduism far outweighs about every religion with its sheer number of observances.

Observances do serve to focus the thoughts of a religion's members—observances like Christmas and Easter, for example. True, both have been commercialized greatly, but at their core both serve to define the Christian religion. The resurrection of Christ at Easter is the defining moment that differentiates Christianity from any other religion—hence the major focus on this specific observance. Many theologians argue that, without the resurrection, the small Christian sect would have faded into obscurity.

However, some of my deepest moments of transcendental experience were not in a strictly spiritual practice but during the period of my life when studying the mystic nature of several religions. More specifically, Jewish mysticism seemed to have the most positive life-altering aspects up to that point in time in my life.

It has been my experience on this journey that spirituality forces a person to confront questions:

- The notion of "me" and my true self
- What are my "*wants*" versus my actual life needs?
- What is the path or way to discover my own purpose in life?
- Meaning in life—is there just one right purpose or direction for someone to follow?

Some of my closest friends have been on a lifetime spiritual journey with no finite answers. Yet, they are overjoyed with the search and would never change a moment of the time they have spent.

Of course, the lines between the two tend to get blurred. I've practiced Buddhism most of my life. It's filled with rituals, beliefs, and endless written text—yet, it is not a religion. Some Buddhist sects in the United States have formal legal churches, but it is my awareness that the formality of being a "Buddhist church" is for the tax incentives, which otherwise are denied to them. Conversely, some of our Protestant sects are rather free flowing, with little directed structure to their services. On the other hand, I have attended spirituality sessions with literally thousands of attendees giving a reasonable argument against the strictly individual nature of the practice.

So, with this lengthy introduction, will my being either spiritual or religious result in weight loss? Probably not as a direct result. Is being spiritual an entry portal to becoming a vegetarian? Not necessarily so. Both of these questions still beg the point as to why worry about spirituality in the reinvention of self?

Embarking on an intentional spiritual journey seems to cement the belief that one person can make a difference. There is a refusal to accept the notion that we are either helpless or simply unable, for some reason, to change because of the actions, beliefs, attitudes, and behaviors of those we encounter. Instead, those on a spiritual path are convinced that the best pathway to achieve change in the attitudes of others is to first change ourselves.

We do live in an age of excess materialism. I have friends who proudly wear a T-shit reading, "Who has the most toys in the end wins."

The use of the goal of spirituality is taken by me in this personal reinvention of self with no second guessing the time and dedication involved. It offers a sense of being beyond material acquisition solely for its own sake. It is a value structure that those I have witnessed on this path live by and helps explain my understanding, why they have lived with joy at the continued seeking involved in spiritual growth.

It is my awareness from reading, study, and attending seminars led by great people, both in the spiritual realm as well as the more traditional religious area, that all have a common base of self-liking. Yes, every major religion and philosophy agree on this basic point. In order to be completely aware and in the moment, both in body and soul, it is important to appreciate, love, respect, and believe in ourselves. With this in mind it seems reasonable to turn our attention to practical or hands-on ways to move forward spiritually. There are several, but it is useful to start with the widely accepted use of meditation.

Meditation as a Vehicle

Thich Nhat Hanh, Zen master, poet, peace activist, and Nobel Prize nominee, tells us the benefits of meditation are being at peace, a positive outlook on life, and personal happiness.

One of the major ways to achieve the above benefits is meditation. Meditation is the roadway for us to increase our skills at being in the present moment. Many theologians argue that the power of both Jesus and Buddha was their ability to stay in the present moment. But let's look at a more contemporary explanation.

I was part of a team that developed a prototype program for vets with posttraumatic stress disorder (PTSD). The program was based on mindfulness training, with meditation as the key path to enhance this skill. Mindfulness allows the mind to stretch the time frame between stimulus and response. For veterans, this "extra" time the decision-making with respect to choices mind now possesses could allow for better decision-making. Decision making the veterans could use when confronted with the issues that cloud their thinking when suffering with PTSD. Instead of possible negative choices like alcohol, drugs, or violence they could, with mindfulness, foresee the negative consequences of these negative choices and pick wiser solutions. Meditation and mindfulness is a widely accepted treatment for PTSD now, with great positive success.

It is the same with eating a diet of healthy food

choices. The knee-jerk response of old junk food habits can be let go in the expanded time awareness to reason out better eating choices. Hence, it's another way for me to achieve sustainable weight-loss goals.

It is the same with relationships. Mindfulness can help expand the mind's horizons to more positive interactions with our fellow humans. I saw this and was the grateful recipient of this at Camp Granola. And on the canoeing trip my initial mistakes were not met with avoidance or rejection by others. No, they were accepted in a nonjudging manner and followed up with helpful, friendly ways to be successful. I was grateful for this and wished to emulate them in my own life's approach to fellow humans.

The process of being in the "moment" changes us and will subsequently change the situation. In my case, it involves seeing myself in a whole new light. Changing our thoughts, especially about our own self, is a big job. Yes, spiritual and religious leaders, as well as many philosophers, agree that we can decide to change our thoughts. Basically, our next breath can take us on the road to become whom we wish to "be."

Spirituality definitions always include points of self-acceptance. Shunryu Suzuki, the Buddhist philosopher and teacher most responsible for the wide acceptance of Buddhism in America, has many quotes but this one always resonated well in my world: "The most important point is to accept yourself and stand on your own two feet."

I cannot remember how many students this quote was shared with over my career as a professor.

The Early Meditation Days

There is the belief that the picture we create of ourselves mentally will manifest into a future self-reality. That was good enough for me to hear. I'd sort of done that to quit smoking many years earlier, and it had worked. No pills, shots, patches, or other over-the-counter aids to quit—just keeping the new vision of self in the forefront of my thoughts. Meditation can be a roadway for implanting the new vision of ourselves in our mind. The new vision for some may be an actual picture, while for others, it may be a feeling. For me, as an auditory person, the new image was more a vocal dialogue in my mind that extolled the positive virtues of this new vision of self. The journey into meditation is more than plopping down and sitting cross-legged.

Yes, the beginning period of meditation can be truly daunting—not daunting from the physical exertion or mental strain. It is the notion of complete stillness and mental nothingness. There was help and valuable coaching over many years with the various trips to Camp Granola, the Zen monastery programs, sessions with Thich Nhat Hanh and attending (TM) Transcendental Meditation classes to name a few. But, at some point, it must come down to putting this idea into personal solitary practice. Sort of like the Nike ads, meaning that reading and going to classes is all good but sooner or later I had to "just do it."

Fortunately, there were friends starting meditation at the same relative time frame and we exchanged experiences and helpful ideas. Breathing and counting breaths is the most common starting point. Breathing is not a daily competition with self to see if today's session could break yesterday's total breath count. No, no. The trick was to just count to some personal pre-agreed total number and then start counting again from the beginning.

The first efforts as an adult at the meditation retreat and with the Zen master as well resulted in having a bad case of the "fidgets" after just a few minutes. Not a great way to start.

As skill levels increased, there were the almost hallucinogenic visions that began to appear. While sharing with other neophytes, we were all convinced it was genuine transcendence that we were experiencing. One friend was convinced there were angels trying, in some manner, to contact him.

Our mentors quickly dismissed these visions we saw in our minds as something to erase, as these were just "mind tricks." The teachers taught us to mentally erase these visions and not get stalled in this entertaining phase, as they referred to it, in our growth experience progression. They instructed us to visualize a chalkboard eraser in our hand and the image on a chalkboard, which we would slowly erase.

As in the case with yoga practice, in meditation, do not eat just before it. Why? Well the body creates gas when converting food for digestion. This gas can and often does exit in an embarrassing manner—not necessairly embarrassing to anyone else other than the person suffering from bloat. The other reason not to eat and meditate is the negative change in blood sugar levels, which can put the meditator to sleep. I cannot count the number of times that has happened to me— especially with the guided meditations led by Tamara Levitt on Calm app. Her voice is the perfect pitch for doing guided meditation, but after a meal, her calming voice has led to a few great but unplanned naps.

Technology has moved into the arena of meditation training. While I have never been to a live meditation training session, where it was recommended to just use the new apps, the apps do have a following. In my training younger people to meditate, the phone apps are resonating well with them and slowly creeping into the daily practice of more senior meditators. Apps include Calm, Headspace, Insight Timer, and Simple Habit to name just a few.

I figured it would be to my advantage to try one of these. And after surfing a number of them—to use a modern term—I selected Calm. It seemed to represent the techno meditation world well enough for me to judge. It allowed for data accumulation of time spent meditating in terms of days, months, and years, as well as actual minutes spent. The time frames to sit for each session varied from ten minutes on up. There were guided selections and others with gentle background sounds or music of the user's choice.

All in all, meditation apps are a great idea for people accustomed to using apps for help with a variety of life's issues. I am now a supporter of these and recommend their use to help people either get started or create and maintain a daily routine. For many meditators my age, there were not options like this when we began the meditation process. The research shows many people above the age of forty-five don't use apps on their phones as much as do younger generations. For those not comfortable with using phone apps, there are wonderful CDs/DVDs with either visual instruction or guided vocal meditations.

It is not the intent here to offer instruction in meditation. There is no lack of options for that. The goal is to present it as a valuable tool to consider for the goal of self-reinvention. It is another piece of the puzzle.

Remember the statistics are not in favor of sustainable weight loss. Let's look at a few of the well-published numbers to drive home the point for selecting a different way to do this:

- Some 45 million people in the United States are dieting on any given day, or from 14 to 36 percent of all adults (Boston Medical Center Health Net).
- In the United States, $33 billion is spent on weight-loss products yearly. That helps explain the preponderance of annoying advertisements.

- Yet, despite the money spent, two-thirds of Americans are overweight or obese (*US News*).
- And according to Penn State University Medical School research, only one in six of those overweight or obese will sustain and maintain weight loss (Penn State University Medical School-Hershey).
- Finally—and I like this silly factoid—the average person spends five weeks, two days, and forty-three minutes on a particular weight-loss diet or plan (Daily Mail.com).

These numbers had changed relatively little over my life. I had clearly been among those bouncing from diet to diet. When the numbers finally sunk in, it opened my eyes to the awareness that more than weight loss needed to be considered. Slowly, my plan emerged, with much trial and error—some humorous as I have shared in the earlier stories. Hopefully, it will not involve others going through the same mistakes and issues.

Let me begin to draw together an outline of a plan with a 360-degree approach in the next chapter.

Recommended Readings

The works recommended here vary from philosophies of positivism and happiness to yoga. Enjoy the eclectic reads.

Kaufman, Barry Neil. *Happiness Is a Choice*. Fawcett Columbine, 1991.

This is a great book that offers us ways to reframe how we look at life and the many issues that come our way almost daily. It offers a protocol of love and compassion that is instantly usable after reading. I so liked the book that I attended programs at the Option Institute started and run by Barry and Suzie Kaufman in Sheffield, Massachusetts.

The Dalai Lama and Howard Cutler. *The Art of Happiness: A Handbook for Living*. New York: Riverhead Books, 1998.

Another great read. For me this book framed happiness as a goal and not something that happens by luck or chance. It is a process that begins with positivism as the guiding philosophy that is linked with gratefulness, which carries us into being in the "now."

CHAPTER 6

The Plan

I'd spent a great deal of time over the years traveling about visiting places like Camp Granola—yes, there were several with very similar ambiance and culture. I'd visited food stores, attended yoga and tai chi seminars, and was also enrolled in classes for them. I'd taken TM meditation training, plus other meditation classes, and had spent countless hours seeking the advice of experts. The time with experts was primarily for nutrition, spirituality, and positive mental reframing and with those who'd successfully reinvented themselves.

During this extended time of "gathering," as it has been referred to by all involved in supporting my quest, I'd been taking notes and mulling about what was the optimum approach. The goal in now organizing this data was to help friends and others with a similar desire in life to shorten the timeline of this process.

My trips to Camp Granola did not stop with one small immersion—of course not. There were many courses and experiences I enrolled in. For example, my friend who accompanied me to the Zen monastery also joined me to spend four days with John Sanford, the famous Episcopal cleric and spirituality writer who was conducting classes at Camp Granola that week. John is a gifted writer, and it was a big push forward for me spiritually to be in this small group session and have the opportunity to listen, question, and provide feedback to this great person about my own thoughts and understanding about spiritual growth.

In another example, my wife and I attended in Washington, DC, the Heart to Heart conference over several years—if memory serves me correctly as to the exact conference name. At these conferences we attended, there was everything from Reiki, to Native American shamans with eagle feathers carrying smudge pots.

For those not familiar with Reiki, it's energy healing therapy. It involves the transfer of universal energy via the palms of the healer's hands. Its origins are from Japan circa the 1800s. During one Reiki session, I sat next to Dennis Weaver of *Gunsmoke* (the Western TV series) fame.

A Native American would do cleansing rituals with an eagle feather and sage smoke from his pot. It was fun to experience so manay different spiritual approaches.

It was an eclectic group, both attending and teaching, who offered a look at so many interesting areas to sample. I did learn how to see and read the auric fields given off by people—that has stayed with me as an aside skill.

Maybe my learning curve is less steep than others, but this type of experiential environment was impactful. Meaning, this path was not a rush job but a glorious learning and an intellectually expanding process.

With this in mind, it is time to offer a broad outline that I would suggest to others. This outline is the culmination of my own lengthy search and was guided by the areas of examination I've presented. Again, remember that this was an evolutionary process that has now been synthesized for presentation to those who have similar life issues and dreams. Failure occurred so often for me in the beginning stages because of short-term goals that centered only on an immediate drop in weight. I understand now that these less-than-satisfying results were a result of not considering a 360-degree strategic approach. The lack of consideration meant I didn't include better health, as well as the intellectual component, through exercise, spiritually broadening my outlook toward life and fellow humanity, eating a diet that supports the overarching strategic goals, and continually maintaining a positive outlook.

The diet selected was as close to a vegetarian modality as possible. Until now, the food items consumed in some past weight-loss-only diets may have shown up in a cardboard box on my doorstep, with little thought given to an active awareness of eating patterns that could be sustainable over an entire lifetime. This is not a criticism of diets supporting this approach, they did help me lose weight. But it displays an answer as to my lack of 360-degree focus irrespective of what diet regimen was tried in the past.

This new look must be a lifestyle change. There is congruence among advisors that this will be a more lengthy process. That notion was expected, given my experience in fostering culture change as a consultant working in various organizations. Radical change, in some instances, can work. But the research shows that what comes off rapidly in weight loss can return just as quickly.

Finally, this and any plan's success is dependent on mindfulness, the moment-to-moment awareness that this is a lifestyle change. Being in the moment allows for making better choices that will lead to success—choices about each of the selected points in such a plan. My plan is a suggestion, and maybe, hopefully, the notion of a broad approach will resonate positively with others. It also means that, if your personal eating choice is food coming in a box, that is just fine but you might also consider the other plan components to up the odds for your success.

The Plan

Let me offer the plan in a bulleted form with more careful examination of each area to follow:

- Daily morning routine
  1. Yoga stretches and positions

2.   Meditation/spiritual growth
3.   Hand weights, exercise bands
- Exercise at gym / health club
- Diet / eating regimen
- Positive mental awareness
- Volunteering / giving back
- Environmental awareness

Yoga

The daily morning ritual is an important item. It certainly is a centering experience, which creates an overall feeling of personal well-being for the rest of the day. Health experts subscribe to the benefits of all three items involved here. It is also a good base set of exercises that help in case life gets in the way and a date at the gym cannot materialize.

The insertion of a yoga part was cemented by an instructor in my hometown with whom I'd enjoyed five years of classes. Her suggestion to me was to give yoga a try before having another surgical procedure. At the time, I was considering back surgery. I've been able to remedy the pain and weakness with decades of a healthy back thanks to her and the daily yoga regimen. Along the way, two torn rotator cuffs and other injuries were able to be remedied with yoga as well. Seeing physical therapists helped me learn new stretches, which were basically other yoga positions.

The therapist did caution that many come to them

for physical therapy, do the required visits, heal, and then quit the exercises. Often the patients would eventually reinjure the same area because it weakened again. So, this routine was for life. Now, I am not advocating that anyone put off his or her physician's recommendations.

This explanation will highlight just a few of the poses used daily and is not intended to be a yoga instruction manual. The dialogue here is for emphasis on areas selected to target my specific physical needs. Targeting is another point of reference for vitamins, as well for specific physical needs. More about targeting in the diet section.

Another caution here is that the poses are but one step in the twelve steps of transcendence in yoga philosophy. The poses are historically used to provide physical flexibility for the mind in the meditation activity that follows the stretches. I am not in that ancient twelve-step program but do find the poses very helpful, both physically and mentally. While traveling in India, I spent a brief stay with a yoga guru master at an ashram, and he was amused that American yoga has morphed into a cardio workout by some US instructors.

The standing part for me is where I begin. I do six stretches and poses just for the shoulders in the standing portion of the yoga morning routine. The standing portion has three additional specific poses used just for enhancing balance. Others are for hamstring, back, side, and neck stretches.

The next poses are in the sitting position, with

stretches that are reminiscent of those taught while I was a member of my high school track team.

This group is followed with lying on my back, with several poses dedicated to hip opening. These are followed by changing to lying on the stomach. This group of poses is helpful for my lower back core area strength and includes the dreaded planks. But, after these, there is the fad favorite downward-facing dog.

Next, are the kneeling positions? While there are several here, two are similar but helpful for those of us who deal with lots of arthritis. The puppy dog pose is where the toes are bent back to offer the flexibility needed to ward off arthritis and contribute to better balance. From puppy dog, it is a simple change to child's pose, where the toes are flattened with weight on my heels and stretching arms forward for the muscles on the side of the chest and upper back.

Before going on to meditation, I will mention that I spent many years with tai chi and found it to be very rewarding, and its health benefits parallel yoga. It is not part of my daily routine, although I do attend special sessions at yoga centers with a close friend who also teaches tai chi. My initial instructor was William C. C. Chen, a master in tai chi from China. If you are a devotee of this health form, feel free to substitute it for yoga.

Meditation

The meditation portion is usually fit in next and can range from ten to thirty minutes. There is no magic in the number of minutes. Even as a child in a Buddhist school in Japan, I recall the emphasis being on the quality of the time spent, not the pure quantity.

Meditation is present in most every religion and philosophy. I taught Christian meditation for a number of years. All of us meditate even when we are unaware of doing so. When I was teaching mindfulness to a class of first-line production supervisors, they were adamant that meditation had never, ever been an experience they'd had. However, when I asked how many fishermen there were, almost all raised their hands. When the comparison between the focus on a fishing bobber and the same discipline in meditation was explained, it became an epiphany for them, and many offered similar life experiences for comparison.

There are many ways to meditate. But the front-runner is breathing. This means to focus on the breath. You can count breaths to some nominal number and restart again. My mentors here often encouraged me to focus on the very brief pause between the in breath and beginning the slow out breath. The pause is almost imperceptible, yet it's there, and the concentration on it drives everything else from the mind. Slow out breath means forming the lips into the shape similar to that for whistling and then to slowly exhale. Panting like my chocolate lab is not the look we're going for in the out breath.

Experts again extol the benefits for breathing emphasis. It clears the lungs, and my pulmonologist reminded me that the added flow of oxygen is a healing therapy for the lungs, as well as for the rest of the body.

During instruction with Thich Nhat Hanh at Camp Granola classes, he regularly used walking meditation. Many people cannot simply sit still. Mindful walking is not a fast pace or like walking the dog. It is awareness of each step on the earth and combined with rhythmic breathing. This combination again requires focus and empties the mind of the mass of nonsense that constantly flows through everyone's brain. That said, I did not "get" mindful walking at first. For me to not comment about everything that passed my view in the lovely woods where we were walking seemed an impossible feat. It took a few times with a mentor to not only appreciate but to look forward to this form of meditation.

The other form of meditation I use as much as breathing while sitting is "loving kindness" meditation. This was learned from Thich Nhat Hanh at another session. It goes like this and is repeated silently in the mind:

> May I be filled with loving kindness,
> May I be well,
> May I be peaceful and at ease,
> May I be happy (Thich Nhat Hanh).

(There are many variants of the above, and also feel free to adjust it to fit your individual circumstance.)

The meditation starts with the above, but the later recitations substitute another person's name. And subsequent recitations continue substituting different names. These can be people who are ill or have some life difficulty; simply friends; and, most difficult but soul cleansing, those you have life difficulty with or even dislike. For example, if it is a woman you wish to extend the blessing of loving kindness to, her name is in the first line and the other lines you insert *she* in place of the *I*.

For those we are in conflict with, it is a positive way to handle anger or disappointment as an alternative to confrontation. For that matter, mentally stewing over this person is not good for anyone's health. For those of Christian persuasion or belief, they are taught to pray for their enemies.

A final point here, if you're routine is to choose a daily prayer segment in lieu of meditation the same wonderful benefits will accrue.

Exercise with Hand Weights

It was later when the hand weights and the exercise bands were included as a regular morning item. Both emerged from having to go to physical therapy. In those sessions, both items were integral to the success of the healing.

It may appear from these examples that I spent a great deal of my free time in therapy. Well, it's not quite that extreme. But in my youth, I did play football and box into college age, and with those two endeavors came three knee surgeries and two ankle surgeries. From mountain biking in the winter snow and cascading down a rocky ledge came other injuries to the shoulders, back, and knees. Believe it or not, in golf I tripped over a wire serving as a fence on a par-three hole to keep carts off the playing surface. That fall resulted in major reconstruction to the left wrist and no golf for eighteen months.

Oh my goodness, it did not seem to be that many surgeries until I typed these examples. I hate to say this, but there were a few more injuries with associated surgeries. Anyway, the point is I have had lots of good coaching for injury recovery, including one longtime therapist who was also well versed in yoga. He was aware of my work interest and incorporated therapy around that discipline.

Hand weights and bands take up little room in the house, making it simple to incorporate them into the morning routine. Mine all fit in a little basket under a straight wooden chair I use for the exercises. Several with weights are for the wrist, and I store a small folding TV table behind the wooden chair for use. All in all, it takes up just a couple of square feet. Plus, the benefits from this form of exercise include keeping bone density at the proper place as we age, while the bands provide great resistance training for tricky body parts like knees, backs, and hips. The different exercises are distributed over the week in an alternating pattern.

These three make up my morning routine, which I do even if I plan later to golf, road bike, or go to the gym for a more intensive cardio workout. Watching a TV show featuring Dr. Oz, where he spoke about a morning routine of his own, I learned that his allegiance to it is much like mine—in that sometimes there is "no time" later in the day for added exercise, and this routine becomes a wonderful balanced plus for the body just by itself.

This routine does take from forty-five to sixty minutes. I just get out of bed that much earlier each day. In the beginning, it was a challenge to forgo the extra bit of sleep or extra time sitting with a cup of coffee. They say it takes three weeks for a new habit to form. It took easily that time period to adjust. But now I cannot imagine a day without this short routine.

Exercise at the Gym

I have discovered that a systematic and simple exercise program works best for me. Many years ago I did try the complex programs at the gym that required me to carry workout sheets on a clipboard so no particular exercise was inadvertently left out. It failed as I am not that attentive to so many different workout details. This self-knowledge triggered a reevaluation of the priorities for the gym days. It came down to needing a simple cardio experience beyond the morning hand weights and bands. Every other gym day is now for exhaustive interval training. The selections of machines were made in consultation with the staff specialist at the gym to target a particular muscle area, which would include a strong cardio element.

Notice again the emphasis on targeting. Well, my target is two fold. The first is cardio for heart health, and the second is for removing a small area of belly fat. It seems my inquiry was met with just a simple nod of the staff specialist's head. Apparently men, as they hit middle age, find the annoying small belly really hard to get rid of. No exception for me either—unfortunately. From his years of education and experience, interval training is the recommended method to remove or significantly decrease belly fat. Of course, I fact-checked him and had to agree.

The days when I am not doing interval training, it's basic cardio workouts. My base is almost always the same two machines. The stationary bike for twenty to thirty minutes and a treadmill for twenty to thirty minutes. These lend themselves to easy use with both cardio training as well as the slightly different interval program. The basic interval training program is to alternate short bursts of very hard biking or treadmill settings followed by reducing the levels to return the heart rate to a lower number and then doing it all over again.

Every age has targeted heart rates to achieve, and the interval training gets to that level. I recommend knowing yours and working in consultation with your health care provider. Modern workout machinery in gyms can easily track heart rates, making the workouts more effective.

Yes, on rare occasions I do use something different machinery wise. It's fun to do that. But it does require more knowledge, as you must learn all the settings on a new type of machine. I have no natural gift for figuring out machines, so this is truly a rare happening for me.

The only other thing included every time at the gym is the big ropes and heavy ball. These thick heavy rope exercises limber up the shoulders and back muscles. For those of us who enjoy road biking, its shoulder strength and flexibility that determine how far and fast the ride will be—not the sore hands and fanny. Again, the ropes are a targeted selection. The ball tossing into what is basically a small trampoline sitting upright at a slight angle helps with coordination and neuro pathway conditioning for reflexes.

The gym time is basically fifty-five minutes to one hour—compact and efficient. It can go beyond when I run into a friend from the past and we gab to catch up about the past years. I do love to see old friends, and in a way, it is therapeutic time for both of us.

Remember, that my mind requires simplicity in the gym, while another person may thrive on the clipboard and many different equipment experiences. If that is your makeup, then it is the correct formula to follow.

There is another recent player in the fitness world that involves the use of an accelerometer to track data and then convert this into measurements. Devices like Fitbit, Apple Watch, Garmin's various devices, and Lintelek, to name just a few, are all used to help track your progress and convert it into usable feedback data. Yet, they are all slightly different. Fitbit's large offering of devices were designed with total emphasis on fitness, and the technology goodies were a bonus. But, Apple Watch, for example, may appear to have the same focus as Fitbit does but comes at it completely different. Apple is first a "smart watch," and the fitness part is the added plus. These devices can track steps, heart rate, and a long laundry list of other items.

Yes, the technology was a lure for me to try. Truthfully, I became obsessed with it and would spend the last minutes before my going to sleep walking around the inside of my house to get the final steps in to achieve my daily step goal. Used more rationally than my own example, research does show these devices can be a helpful in achieving the overarching goal of personal and physical transformation.

No, I never lost any weight with using one. As I have evolved my goals and plans, any of these fine products could now fit into the scheme and be held in check as not to become an obsessive negative. Mental game playing came much too readily for me, and I became a master at achieving "steps" in a questionable manner. For example, there is a rocker in my den, and I would fasten the device to the chair's front bottom area so the rocking motion while involved in my daily reading would record steps.

One final note here—the ten thousand daily step goal did not originate out of any systematic research. It is a marketing idea, and the origination of counting steps with devices goes back to Japan decades before Fitbit was even a product for sale.

So much for exercise. On to the tricky eating part.

The Eating Part

With the initial goal to become one of the beautiful people, eating—or better said, what to eat—becomes important. By now, the picture is clear for me that following the latest fad diet will not work long term. The weight does come off. However, it's in the transition from the fad diet to real life where the difficulty always arises. Most fad diets are like events in isolation away from the day to day need to eat after the weight loss part is accomplished. For me to claim a successful eating transition back to the reality of normal meals was questionable, especially when the whole program to lose weight was food delivered in a box or bought at the local diet franchise owner's store or purchased in frozen packages at the food store. The time came for me to step back and examine this notion of what-to-eat in more detail.

Earlier I discussed meeting with the various nutritionists over the years, reading lots of material on proper eating, and speaking with acquaintances who'd successfully kept the weight off bt making the transition to normal life eating. This wealth of information helped me to decide the path I would take.

Now, normal life eating is not to be confused with poor food selection. Normal eating is your plate at dinnertime seated at the table with the rest of the family containing very close to or the same food—meaning that no one there is eating a very unhealthy meal, and my decisions have impacted the other members of the family to move toward wiser selections.

The notion that a family all sits at the same table eating together is part of the problem for many obese individuals. The number of families sharing common meal times has continually diminished over the past decades, to be replaced by less healthy, fast, or convenient foods from outside the home and consumed as an individual. But that is another issues we hope to tackle by finding our own particular eating regimen that will preclude unhealthy food choices.

It is worth noting that any rapid weight loss program has associated health risks. In the most sever cases rapid weight loss can be addictive leading people into eating disordered behaviors. One diagnosis is called 'atypical anorexia' where a person has the same experiences and behaviors such as starvation and mental issues like a person with anorexia. Yet, in the atypical anoxeria case the person is not clinically underweight. In addition our society glorifies the very slender people in commercial ads and in subtel inference in TV porograming. This contributes too many psychological and health related issues among many young people. It is another reason to foster a more balanced approach that involves a lifestyle adoption to a sustainable and healthy approach to this aspect of life.

My personal choice is to move very close to being a vegetarian. That immediately raised many conflicting arguments about getting enough protein and vitamin B12.

As an aside, it also included many questions as to why this hybrid choice. Here is the somewhat short answer to that legitimate question. First, it takes a lot of careful planning to balance amino acids, and I am a low-maintenance type person. Four ounces of fish, eggs, cheese, or chicken per week can handle these two issues. Secondly, I did try vegetarian eating for eight years, and aside from the fact that only modest weight loss was registered, the overabundance of fiber was too much for my body. Talk about bloating. Finally, it is not an ideological philosophy for me but a choice to achieve a healthier life. If I visit a friend's home, and the friend has proudly crafted a bacon, cheese, and broccoli quiche for dinner, there will be no refusing it. I simply limit the portion size.

So, on to the protein arguments. One well-versed friend still felt the four ounces may be too little. Despite all the articles abounding on this topic—*healthy eating means healthy food choices*—it is still a difficult concept for many to grasp. These choices must still include protein. The research seems to indicate that for men more than women protein mentally is equated with meat. There are other foods where this key body nutrient is contained. I am not a bodybuilder where more protein is part of the success equation.

A word of caution about upping the protein portion above the suggested 15 percent of total caloric input range to the 25 percent range typically found in high-protein diets is necessary. The red flag of caution is primarily waved if there are kidney issues. If so, then seek the approval of a specialists before starting. Similarly, upping the protein range just from beef in a diet brings on the inconclusive arguments about cardiovascular issues. Again, consult your cardiologist if there are possible heart/vascular issues.

With today's abundant new food options, I can have minimal animal protein thanks to vegetable isolates like pea protein. Impossible Burgers and Beyond Beef are just two of the popular brands formed to look and taste like beef. And these same proteins are available as dairy milk substitutes.

Any trip to the once sacred dairy section containing milk is a new experience for the uninitiated. There are literally a dozen different substitutes for traditional dairy milk with all containing calcium, protein, and Vitamin D. They range from almond to pea, oat, and soy, to name just a few.

As you can quickly see, the pulling together of an eating plan will be no easy feat. At the end of this chapter there is an article link to examine the hazards of high-protein diets. But there are similar warnings for any substitution diet that eliminates one of the three food groups.

Let's stay with the notion of complexity and look for a moment at planning a diet if there are more severe kidney issues like stage 3 kidney disease. Now, the hope of becoming a vegetarian has the complexity game taken to a new and more challenging level. Old standbys like broccoli, for example, have too much phosphorus contained in them.

The foods to *avoid* short list includes pretzels (a favorite of mine); chips, dips, and avocados; all canned foods; whole grains including whole wheat bread and brown rice; bananas; dairy products, oranges and orange juice; pickles, olives, and relish; apricots; potatoes and sweet potatoes; tomatoes, premade meals; spinach; beets; and dates, raisins, and prunes. Talk about planning challenges for pulling together a meal that will taste good—this avoid list is daunting.

The okay to eat list includes blueberries, garlic, olive oil, skinless chicken breast, cranberries, red or black grapes (not white or green), pineapple, all colors of bell peppers, and cauliflower. In the grains list are buckwheat (it is not a regular grain since it is in the rhubarb family), pearled barley, and couscous. This is daunting in the mere shortness of the options.

Now, there are items like eggs that can be used in moderation or as egg whites. These additions are recommended after the creatinine blood levels are at least stabilized. Many traditional as well as homeopathic physicians ascribe to the belief that proper eating is the preferred highway for the body to heal itself. Individuals with stage 3 kidney disease who have kept to the list of accepted eating in a fairly rigorous manner have reported delays for the onset of serious kidney disease treatments and ramifications.

The goal here is not to cover all possible negative health issues but to offer an example that, even if someone is facing the above issue or perhaps something like diabetes, the 360-degree option to self-reinvention does not preclude his or her participation.

My Personal Eating Regimen

My own eating regimen is not to be taken as what everyone or anyone else should elect to follow. With all the background work, this seems to work for me. With that disclaimer, here is what I follow:

Breakfast, about four mornings a week, is a small bowl of sunflower and pumpkin seeds, dried cranberries or tart cherries (no-sugar varieties when available), and chopped walnuts. For variety, this combination may be mixed with yogurt. About two mornings a week, it is a fruit and vegetable smoothie with yogurt and protein drink added to the blender/juicer. The fruits and vegetables vary with what is fresh and available in my pantry. This leaves one morning a week where the breakfast is at a meeting and the menu is out of my control or when I am too tired or lazy to do anything but sip tea for the morning meal.

Lunch is typically the big meal of the day when possible. We all know about best-laid plans in life.

Life often gets in the way of this eating order, where the noon meal is the primary feast of the day. When possible, it is a meal made up of vegetables and soup (my eastern European heritage elevates soup to an unrealistically high level of respect). The vegetables are cooked according to many tasty recipes learned from mentors and coaches. Often, these meals contain one of the meat substitutes. The notion here is that the lunch meal has more time for digestion than one eaten later in the day.

Dinner—the later meal—ranges from the basic bowl of cereal to a fancy, medium-sized salad with a balsamic dressing. Another regular meal is a cup of soup with a sugar free Jell-O. Again, life gets in the way at least two nights a week, being out with friends or attending business dinners, family events, and the "whatevers" of life. When this happens, I try to use as much restraint as possible.

The other goal is to not snack or eat for the next fourteen hours after dinner. This is not possible on those two nights a week where dinner may not start till 8:00 or 9:00 p.m. This pause in eating has recently become a "fad diet" of its own. Called the IF (interval fasting) diet plan or some name similar to this, it involve pausing eating over some specified time period. I did not know it had become a new diet fad since my nutritionist recommended it a decade before it hit the best-seller list. The biggest selling point is—you guessed it—yes, weight loss. Secondary benefits include better insulin sensitivity. Insulin control is a plus for those with type 2 diabetes and those wishing to lower cholesterol.

The notion expressed with the IF option is the body has its own internal digestion clock. It is referred to as circadian rhythm. This says that eating during the busy hours of the day helps metabolize food more efficiently. This translates to lower blood sugar and better lipids, which include cholesterol and triglycerides.

To be honest, I did not start the fasting because of the above. My motives were simple and basic and included better sleep—a full stomach from a big evening meal is hard on many of us sleep wise—and to reduce inflammation. Inflammation is an issue for arthritis, joint pain, and coronary disease prevention. I entered this fad through the back door—meaning I was already actively involved when the best sellers and numerous articles about it appeared on the newsstands. It felt nice to be ahead of the curve for once.

The idea of no hard pretzels as a nighttime snack was a big deal for me to get over. Most junk food has never been on my want list, so bragging about leaving them behind would be false. During the first three days of fasting at night, my stomach would start growling about 9:00 p.m. and not quit till morning.

Positive Mental Attitude

"The path into the light seems dark, the path forward seems to go back, the direct path seems long, true power seems weak, true purity seems tarnished, true

steadfastness seems changeable, true
clarity seems obscure, the greatest art
seems unsophisticated, the greatest love
seems indifferent, the greatest wisdom
seems childlike."

—Tao Te Ching

The choice of the above quote helps set the stage for including positivism as a 360-degree item in my reinvention of self. This area has some fine lines of difference in thought and personal actions from spirituality. Both have dramatically altered my life. Positive mental reframing of life's challenges is a skill set fundamental to sustainable personal happiness.

Life presents a seemingly endless onslaught of challenges—so many at times that parking our attitudes in a negative framework seems the easier route. There is no arguing that being negative is easier. Yet, the psychological and medical research supports that a positive mental attitude is associated with better health, longevity, improved relationships, and even facial muscle memory that supports a more attractive look. With all that and more going for it, why is it so hard?

The difficulty with being positive or upbeat is not new. A cursory look at history reveals it does show up all through time. I sent a note to a biblical scholar friend asking about positivism in the Bible. The response was dozens of biblical citations that refer to or discuss the notion of positivism. I did ask why not the exact word and was quickly informed that it was Auguste Comte, the French philosopher, who coined the term *positivism* in the early nineteenth century. No such word was available in early times.

But the real father of modern-day positivism is Norman Vincent Peale. For those of us who dream of being successful writers, Peale's best-selling book of 1952, *The Power of Positive Thinking*, was on the best-seller list for 186 consecutive weeks and sold 5 million copies. The Dutch reformed minister died in 1993 at the age of ninety-five. His career as a minister began with the Methodist church but later switched when he started his own Protestant-based faith church.

What is amazing to me is the heavy criticism he suffered when the book was first published. This critics basically felt Peale was trying to get his readers to flee negative thoughts, and many critics lumped negativity in with the notion of evil. In current thought by many, Peale is looked at as reframing negativity into positive actions and thoughts, and the notion of evil is dropped from this discussion.

More currently, there's Robert Schuller, the famous clergyman associated with positivism and the Crystal Cathedral, plus the *Hour of Power*, a weekly TV program broadcast from the cathedral. Schuller taught self-belief and was referred to as an apostle of positive thinking. Later, Ken Blanchard, author of the best seller *The One Minute Manager* and situational leadership theory, used positivism as a roadway to successful leadership, as well as life skills in general.

How does someone stop griping and be positive? Is this some kind of unreal world that positivism asks the user to believe in? The answer to the first question implies that we are in a constant state of seeking mindfulness in the present moment. We're aware of our interactions with others and reframing our responses to negative situations presented to us. This does not mean that bad things will never come our way. That would be a fantasy world. But we have the ultimate power of choice in how we respond.

Yes, the word used was *power*, and it is an assertive skill to be positive. To not let events that are out of our control dictate our happiness is power. It's the crux of PTSD mindfulness training for vets and others like emergency room personnel. It's expanding the horizon of opportunities from which to respond and deciding not to select a choice that will lead to a negative self-consequence. There is no greater power than selecting how you and I choose to respond.

Barry Neil Kauffman's best seller, *Happiness Is a Choice*, goes to the heart of choices we all can make when faced with any sort of adversity in life. The nice part of choosing a positive thinking life philosophy is because this is not something where some advanced training or university degree is required. It is my awareness that our next breath can take us to become the kind of positive and loving people we want to be, and it's inherent within all of us.

Volunteering

I was fortunate to grow up in a home where giving back was a natural part of life. It was never a celebrated event, just the expected behavior. My father taught that if we as citizens expected to live in a positive, healthy society, then contributing to its success was required.

I have spent my career working in an intellectual environment, and for many in that world, their sophisticated complaints and griping are their "doing." Let's be clear about this, arguing among ourselves and mutually supported griping is *not* doing something about the conditions in life we do not agree with.

The big hurdle here is to examine where your passion lies. There is no lack of places for people to volunteer their talents.

There are numerous studies that support the health benefits of helping those in need—from lower blood pressure, reduced stress, and better sleep to a more positive attitude and a sense of inner peace. From the science of weight loss, lowering stress will reduce cortisol levels, which will reduce fat buildup. Cortisol is present in most of our body cells, and that fact alone supports its dramatic effect on issues of our overall health. It helps control blood sugar levels—a good thing for diabetics or prediabetics—contributes to regulating metabolism; decreases inflammation; and balances the salt-to-water levels in the body, which affects blood pressure levels. Yes, all that positive health goodness from offering a few hours of time at the local soup kitchen—or wherever.

Volunteering fits nicely into the 360-degree rebuild of a total person.

Environmental Awareness

This is not a forum to argue global climate change. Other books do that very well. Environmental awareness is a moment-to-moment awareness of how we all affect the earth by our string of daily choices. A close friend is a role model for me and others by his daily choices to not use disposable plastic water bottles or disposable coffee pods for his morning cup and to select an environmentally friendly car to drive. Daily environmentally positive choices by each of us acting individually will make a difference. I still wince at my childhood lack of environmental understanding, when I would toss an empty can into a bush to dispose of it instead of walking to a trash can. Thanks to being a Boy Scout, where they teach environmentally responsible behavior, the message was learned by me at an early age.

Ever since I was a small child, I observed my mother recycle cans, bottles, paper, and old clothes, along with a host of additional items for use by those less fortunate. Her model behavoir was absorbed by me as I aged and made me acutely aware of living on a finite planet with limited resources that needed to be shared by all and respected for all its living inhabitants. Environmental awareness could well have been under the umbrella of volunteering, as it is a form of giving back to the planet and our fellow inhabitants.

This also became an early pathway for me to cross over to whom I wished to become. The people I admired most also possessed a similar sense of earth awareness. This practice offers very similar health benefits to volunteering. It also fosters a stronger awareness of self-esteem from walking the path in a positive manner.

Reading Doris Longacre's *Living More with Less* was an eye-opening experience as to all the ways any person could easily incorporate this practice into his or her life. Supported by the Mennonites, the Longacre's book gives practical ways of living with less. The Mennonites are hands-on volunteers with feet on the ground in times of emergencies. The ideas in the book are ways for all of us to reduce our impact on the earth.

The points of this plan to reinvent myself is very singular in nature. Others who have embarked on similar journeys picked slightly different notions to focus upon. I am surprised at the similarities of overall content among those of us who become seekers of the path and by others whom have published similar works. The joy is in the journey, and the final destination is always a work in progress.

Let's now move on to give a score card of sorts about this quest of mine.

Recommended Reading

In previous chapters, I mentioned Barry Neil Kauffman's *Happiness is a Choice* and Norman Vincent Peal's book on positivism, so they will not be repeated here. But the eclectic nature of these suggestions will be fun reading if you have not looked at some of these already.

Feuerstein, George. *The Yoga Tradition: Its History, Literature, Philosophy and Practice.* Prescott, Arizona: Hohm Press, 2001.

The title alone gives some idea as to the comprehensive nature of the work. After reading this several times, I felt as if I had finished a graduate program in yoga. It has always been a pet peeve of mine that so many "certified" yoga instructors' knowledge pretty much starts and ends with their grasp of the various positions. Yet yoga is so much more.

Ken Wilber wrote the foreword and sums up the difference between the view of the yoga scholar and the view of the practioner. Ken is one of the most brilliant thinkers of our time.

Kornfield, Jack. *A Path with a Heart: A Guide through the Perils and Promises of Spiritual Life.* New York: Bantam Books, 1993.

Kornfield, Jack. *After the Ecstasy, the Laundry.* Bantam Books, 2000.

The above two suggested books are by Jack Kornfield. I suggest reading them in the order presented, as the second does build on the first. They are witty and funny yet offer great wisdom on both spiritualty and Buddhism

Longacre, Doris Janzen. *Living More with Less.* Scottdale, PA: Herald Press, 1980.

The book was discussed within this chapter. It is a timeless book with a mountain of ideas.

CHAPTER 7

The Scorecard

Let me give my "report card" about this journey. The book opens with the humorous story from Camp Granola many decades earlier. Although I have returned there often, I still shake my head at the difficult start of my journey. Fortunately, the staff at these camps do turn over, so there are no lingering members to tell the tale of my beginnings.

A very important point that was driven home to me in this quest was that being in the moment is a constant way of life. It is not reserved for special occasions, such as teaching veterans suffering from posttraumatic stress disorder (PTSD) about mindfulness. Mindfulness becomes a way of life. Every one of the six areas of this plan are more successfully approached from a moment-to-moment awareness.

The big question for some might be, did it all result in losing weight and keeping it off? The short answer is yes. Slightly over fifty pounds were lost and remained off for eleven years. So far.

Now, I did take off more—about ten more pounds. But that ten pounds is a yo-yo for me. The period from Thanksgiving through Christmas is tough, and I regain that ten. Winter is not my friend, as I do not exercise outside when the temperature is below fifty degrees. Kind of wimpy, but being cold is the worst feeling in the world for me. So why invite it into one's conscious awareness? With spring and vigorous outside activity, this ten always goes away.

However, now the ten must go along with ten more. It is a genetic heart thing, where weight loss is a real positive. Is it necessary to redo my entire personal plan? No. All that will be done here is tweaking the eating part to include foods to now avoid—meaning, the new changes will be absorbed into the plan as the new normal. As of this writing, five pounds are already off, but these are in the yo-yo range of the ten pounds, so they really don't count.

The next big question posed is, Am I part of the beautiful people? Well, beauty is in the mind/eye of the beholder—an old axiom but so true. As a former linebacker and boxer, beauty in the classic sense is not a realistic feat. But my current vision of self is not based on the narrow definitions I originally started with. In the 360-degree approach, there are multiple looks that define myself and others trying this plan in a healthier manner, both physically and mentally. Being in the present moment stretches the arena of thought between stimulus and response. This gift allows anyone to take back the self-power to decide to like and love him or herself in this moment. If someone is following his or her own plan of self-reinvention, there are many reasons beyond the numbers on a bathroom scale to love oneself. When I quit smoking decades ago, it was a new self-image that won the day, enabling this unhealthy habit to disappear.

I opened my picture album. Yes, it is an old-fashioned one with actual paper pictures. I love this type versus electronic ones because I can write the names of everyone in a group shot, along with other notes for instant memory recall. There, in all the group shots, contained the pictures of those I felt were beautiful people. In reality they are simply people. They're people just like me—people who, in their case, had consciously achieved a broad comprehension of the areas now in the plan I follow. These were not photos of perfect models ready for a photo shoot—just great people who'd accepted and helped me along the way.

It has been a point of pride that I have helped mentor others in meditation, to try tai chi or yoga, to lend their talents to a nonprofit, and to understand and respect the environment. This is not some unchangeable mandate to follow. The nature of change itself is a fluid concept. The passage of time and circumstance also drive change. For example, my fourth knee surgery was a partial knee replacement. It was a success, yet even after eighteen months, there are some yoga positions that must be modified and some that must be eliminated. New ones will be added to compensate for their loss, but I will still achieve the goals—just with new positions. Knee surgery is not a major life changer, but it illustrates that yoga keeps the mind flexible in order to more readily accept changes. The plan allows for an easy incorporation of these while staying on the path.

I do hope the stories and struggles on my part were helpful, as well as a bit humorous. The goal was to impart a way to halt everything from self-doubt and frustration to self-loathing in the weight-loss process. And it was to help all the readers know that a one-dimensional look focusing on just weight loss becomes a self-limiting strategy from the very start.

AUTHOR'S NOTES

During the final stages of writing this book a whole new challenge emerged-Coronavirus (COVID-19). The eating part became a challenge to find food stores where the fresh items I enjoy in the process were still available. In a strange way the social distincing and the lock down helped focus my attention on completing the book. Honestly, it became a challenge for me to become disciplined and not to snack from boredom.

There are just too many people to actually name to thank for their help and support. Many will see themselves in the various chapters. My wife does deserve recognition as someone who put up with my countless diets, eating fads, and a virtual library of cookbooks and best sellers expounding on the latest fads. She is also the genius behind my learning how to acquire a new self-image. She has two masters and doctoral studies in health and was a vast resourse of knowledge in pulling together this material.

The places visited are real. Camp Granola exists— just not under that name—as do many of the other places mentioned. It was easier to simply not name them than to seek out the permissions. I have no doubt they would have been granted, so the fault rests with me.

My thanks to the research librarians at Penn State University, Mont Alto, and at Shippensburg University for their help over the many years in finding the books and articles that helped guide my search.

Similarly, my thanks go to my nutritionist and physician friends who spent time with me going over countless blood tests and other results to judge my progress. Yes, I am a data geek who carefully documented eating, vitamins, herbs, exercise, and other changes to key blood level indicators of success.

The components of cholesterol are an example of where my monitoring vitamin and herbal inputs took my cholesterol from the 230-plus range to 119 without the use of prescribed pharmaceuticals—part of my targeting approach to problems. I am not opposed to prescribed medicines and will use them when absolutely necessary. But all medicines run through the kidneys and liver, which, over the long term, affects those organs.

This process was carefully journaled. I have journaled all my life, so this was no hardship. It made for instant recall of events. If simple storytelling were the goal of the book, it would be several volumes long.

Printed in the United States
By Bookmasters